Phone Numbers

Hospital name: _____

    Phone: _____

    Address: _____

Taxi phone: _____

Dentist's name: _____

    Phone: _____

    Address: _____

Other medical phone numbers:

_____

_____

_____

_____

Mom's work phone: _____

Dad's work phone : _____

Family member's name: _____

    Phone: _____

Babysitter's name: _____

    Phone: _____

Neighbor's name: _____

    Phone: _____

Neighbor's name: _____

    Phone: _____

Other phone numbers:

_____

_____

What To Do When You're Having a Baby

Easy to Read • Easy to Use

Gloria Mayer, R.N.
Ann Kuklierus, R.N.

Institute for Healthcare Advancement
501 S. Idaho Street, Suite 300
La Habra, California 90631
(800) 434-4633

© 2011 Institute for Healthcare Advancement
501 S. Idaho Street, Suite 300
La Habra, California 90631
(800) 434-4633

Library of Congress Cataloging-in-Publication Data
Mayer, Gloria G.
  What to do when you're having a baby : easy to read - easy to use /
Gloria Mayer, Ann Kuklierus.
      p. cm.
  ISBN 978-0-9701245-6-2 (pbk. : alk. paper)
 1. Pregnancy. 2. Childbirth. I. Kuklierus, Ann. II. Title.
  RG525.M137 2004
  618.2—dc22

                                                    2004008840

Printed in the United States
13 12 11   16 15 14
ISBN: 978-0-9701245-6-2

To Our Readers

Pregnancy is an exciting time in a woman's life. You will notice many changes in your body and how you feel. You may wonder if these changes are normal. This book will answer many questions. It will tell you:

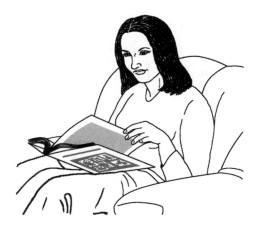

- What you need to do to have a healthy baby.
- Things that can hurt you and your baby.
- Body changes that happen in pregnancy.
- What you can do to feel better.

This book was written to help you have a healthy baby. It gives you a month by month guide to your pregnancy. It tells you how big your baby is each month and how your baby looks. It also explains some of the discomforts you may have and what you can do for them.

This book does not take the place of getting health care throughout your pregnancy. See your doctor often. Some women use a nurse midwife instead of a doctor for normal pregnancy.

To Our Readers

Here are some things to do when you get this book:

- Fill in the phone numbers at the front of this book. Keep this book where it is easy to find.

- Turn to pages x–xii to find out what's in this book.

- Turn to pages viii–ix for a list of things that are not normal. Call your doctor or nurse right away if you get any of these signs.

- Read about things that can hurt your baby on pages 14–18.

- Read about what you need to eat to have a healthy baby (see pages 25–29).

- Learn about the changes you and your baby have every month. Read about each month so you will know what to expect (see pages 38–83).

- See the word list at the back of the book. It gives the meaning of some words in the book.

This book was read by doctors and nurses who work with pregnant women like you. They agree with the information in this book. They feel it is safe and helpful.

Each woman is different. Some things in this book may not be right for you. If you have questions or concerns, call your doctor or nurse right away. Always do what your doctor or nurse tells you.

My Doctor Visits

Day / Date	Time	My Weight
_____	_____	_____
_____	_____	_____
_____	_____	_____
_____	_____	_____
_____	_____	_____
_____	_____	_____
_____	_____	_____
_____	_____	_____
_____	_____	_____
_____	_____	_____
_____	_____	_____
_____	_____	_____
_____	_____	_____
_____	_____	_____

When to Get Help Right Away

Your body goes through many changes during pregnancy. Most of these changes are normal. Some changes are not OK. They are called warning signs. Call your doctor or nurse right away if you have any of these warning signs:

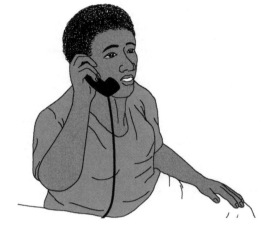

- Bleeding from your vagina
- Gush of water or fluid leaking from your vagina
- Discharge from your vagina that does not seem normal. It can smell, burn or itch.
- Sharp pains in your belly
- Very bad throwing up. You can't keep down any food or fluids for 24 hours.
- Cramps that feel like you're having a period
- Dull lower back pain. It is not the same as your normal backache. It comes and goes.
- Pressure in your lower belly. It feels like your baby is pushing down.
- A feeling like your baby is balling up inside of you
- Your baby moves less than before or not at all.

When to Get Help Right Away

- Your uterus starts to tighten (feel hard). This happens every 10–15 minutes or more often. This is called having contractions.
- Your vision is blurred or you see spots.
- You have swelling in your face or hands.
- You feel very dizzy or faint.
- You have constant or very bad headaches.
- You fall or were in an accident.
- You have a fever of 100.6 degrees F or higher.
- You have chills.
- You have pain or burning when you pee.

Call your doctor or nurse anytime you think something may be wrong. Do not be afraid to ask your doctor if what you are feeling is OK.

What's in This Book

What's in This Book

Getting Ready to Have a Baby

1

Notes

Before You Get Pregnant

What is it?

It is when you decide you want to have a baby. You are not pregnant yet, or you may be pregnant and not know it.

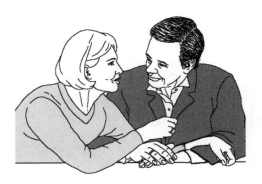

What do I need to know?

- When you stop using birth control, you need to start taking care of your health. You can get pregnant and not know it.

- A healthy woman is more likely to have a healthy baby.

- Some things you do before you get pregnant can help your baby.

- Folic acid is a B vitamin. It protects unborn babies from some birth defects. A woman planning to get pregnant needs to take a vitamin with 400 mcg of folic acid every day. It is hard to get all the folic acid you need from food.

- Women need to get 1000 mcg of folic acid during pregnancy. You can get this amount by taking vitamins and eating foods high in folic acid.

- Here's a list of foods high in folic acid:
  - Dark green leafy vegetables like spinach and lettuce
  - Broccoli and asparagus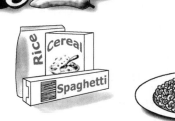
  - Oranges, pineapples, cantaloupes, bananas, and avocados
  - Cereal, pasta, and rice with folic acid added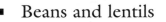
  - Beans and lentils
- Some fish have a lot of mercury, which can harm an unborn baby. Women trying to get pregnant and pregnant women should not eat more than 12 ounces of fish a week. They should eat fish low in mercury like shrimp, salmon, or canned light tuna. Women should not eat fish high in mercury like shark, swordfish, tilefish, king mackerel, or albacore tuna.
- Very thin women have a higher risk of having a small baby. They need to gain some weight before getting pregnant.
- Heavy women can get diabetes and high blood pressure during pregnancy. They need to lose weight before getting pregnant.
- Some women may need to get shots and medical tests before getting pregnant.

- Women who have health problems like diabetes or high blood pressure need to see their doctor before getting pregnant. They may be at risk for having a baby with problems.

What should I do?

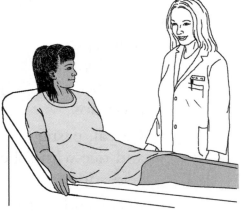

- Go to a doctor even if you feel well. Tell the doctor that you want to have a baby. Your doctor may give you an exam and do some tests.

- Tell your doctor about any sickness you had in the past. Be honest with your doctor.

- Get tested for sexually transmitted diseases (STDs) and for HIV. If you have an STD, you need to get treated before you get pregnant.

- Tell your doctor about all the medicines you take. This includes medicines doctors ordered for you and things you buy at the store, like vitamins and herbs.

- Tell your doctor if you take street drugs, even if you do it only a few times a month.

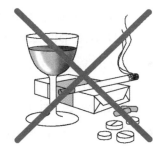

- Stop smoking, drinking alcohol, and taking street drugs. Ask your doctor to help you stop.

- Stop taking birth control pills 3 months before you want to get pregnant. Use a condom for birth control during the 3 months.

- Eat foods high in folic acid listed on page 3.

- Take a vitamin every day with folate or folic acid. Ask your doctor which vitamin to take. It's hard to get enough folic acid from food alone.

- Do not eat more than 12 ounces of fish a week. Don't eat fish high in mercury like shark, swordfish, tilefish, king mackerel, or albacore tuna.

- If you are heavy, talk to your doctor about diet and exercise. You need to lose weight before you get pregnant. It's not safe to diet when you are pregnant.

- If you are very thin, you need to gain some weight before you get pregnant. Your doctor can help you.

- Keep your teeth and gums healthy. Brush your teeth with a soft toothbrush. Do this after every meal and at bedtime. Floss your teeth every day. See a dentist for a check-up every six months.

When do I call my doctor or nurse?

- Call if you want to get pregnant.
- Call as soon as you think you are pregnant.
- Call if you have questions about getting pregnant.
- Call the National Drug and Alcohol Treatment hotline if you need help to stop using alcohol or drugs. Their number is 1-800-662-4357. You can also find a place for help by looking in the front of the phone book under Alcohol and Drug Abuse.

Signs of Pregnancy and What Happens in Your Body

What is it?

Pregnancy happens when a man's sperm meets (fertilizes) a woman's egg after sex. The fertilized egg attaches to the wall of the uterus and grows into a baby.

Here are the parts of the body you need to know.

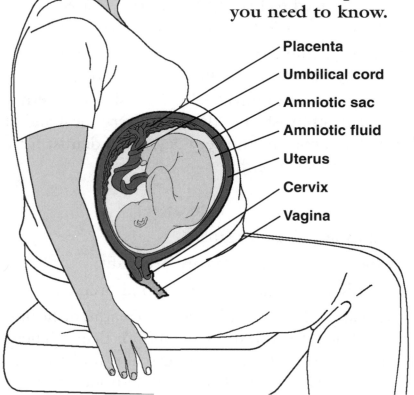

Placenta

Umbilical cord

Amniotic sac

Amniotic fluid

Uterus

Cervix

Vagina

Uterus or Womb
(YOU-ter-us or WOOM)

This is the part of your body that carries a growing baby. The muscles of the uterus stretch as the baby grows.

Amniotic Sac
(am-nee-AW-tic sak)

It is like a bag that grows inside the uterus. It holds the baby, the placenta, and a watery fluid called amniotic fluid. It is often called the bag of water. It protects the growing baby inside the uterus.

Placenta
(pluh-SEN-tuh)

It grows in the uterus of a pregnant woman. It supplies the baby with food and air. It is attached to the baby by the umbilical cord. The placenta comes out after the baby is born. It is also called the afterbirth.

Umbilical Cord
(um-BILL-ih-cal cord)

It connects the baby to the placenta. The cord brings food to the baby from the mother through the placenta. It takes away waste from the baby. The umbilical cord is cut after the baby is born. The baby doesn't feel it. The part left on the baby becomes the belly button.

Cervix

(SIR-viks)

It is the lower end or neck of the uterus. It opens into the vagina. The cervix opens wide during labor to let the baby out.

Vagina

(vuh-JIE-nuh)

It is the last passage that the baby goes through during birth.

What do I need to know?

- Here are some early signs of pregnancy:
  - Missing your monthly period
  - Sore breasts
  - Feeling sick to your stomach and throwing up (also called morning sickness)
  - Wanting certain foods (also called food cravings)
  - Needing to pee often
  - Feeling tired
- Some women have one or more early signs. Some women do not have any early signs. They even have a light period in the first month.
- The first months of pregnancy are very important to your baby's health. Women should not take any drugs, smoke, or drink alcohol. These things can hurt the baby for life.

- A woman can get pregnant even if she is using birth control.

- A woman does not know when she will get pregnant. Some women get pregnant as soon as they stop using birth control and have sex. It takes longer for other women. It can take up to 1 year.

- Once a woman decides to have a baby, she needs to start taking care of herself as if she is pregnant. She should start taking vitamins with folic acid.

- Women can buy a home pregnancy test to find out if they are pregnant. They can also get a pregnancy test at a doctor's office or a health clinic.

What should I do?

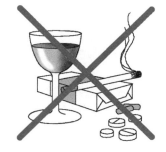

- Do not use drugs, drink alcohol, or smoke if you are trying to get pregnant. These things can harm your baby for life.

- Do not take any medicines unless your doctor says it's OK. This includes medicines you buy and medicines ordered by other doctors.

- Call your doctor if you think you may be pregnant. Your doctor will do a test to find out if you are pregnant.

- Your doctor may do a pelvic exam and check your uterus.

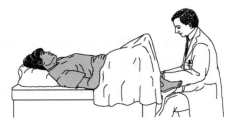

When do I call my doctor or nurse?

- Call if you want to have a baby.
- Call if you think you may be pregnant.

Warning Signs and When to Call Your Doctor

What is it?

It's things that you feel or see that are not normal.

What do I need to know?

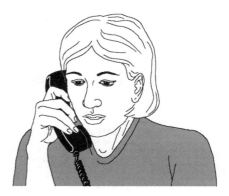

- Most women who take care of their health have healthy pregnancies.

- A woman's body goes through many changes during pregnancy. Most of the changes are normal.

- Some changes are not OK. They are signs that something is wrong. These are called warning signs.

- Here's a list of warning signs. Call your doctor or nurse right away if you have any of these signs:

  - Bleeding from your vagina

  - Gush of water or fluid leaking from your vagina

  - Discharge from your vagina that does not seem normal

  - Sharp pains in your belly

  - Very bad throwing up. You can't keep down any food or fluids for 24 hours.

  - Cramps that feel like you're having a period

  - Dull lower back pain. It is not the same as your normal backache. It comes and goes.

- Pressure in your lower belly. It feels like your baby is pushing down.
- A feeling like your baby is balling up inside of you
- Your baby moves less than before or not at all.
- Your uterus starts to tighten (feel hard). This happens every 10–15 minutes or more often. This is called having contractions.
- Your vision is blurred or you see spots.
- You feel very dizzy or faint.
- You have swelling in your face or hands.
- You have constant or very bad headaches.
- You fall, were in an accident, or were hurt by someone.
- You have a fever of 100.6 degrees F or higher.
- You have chills.
- You have pain or burning when you pee.

- Many problems can be treated if you get medical help right away.

What should I do?

- Know the warning signs listed above.
- Call your doctor right away if you are having any warning signs.

When do I call my doctor or nurse?

- Call if you have one or more warning signs.
- Call if you think something may be wrong. Do not be afraid to ask if what you are feeling is normal.

Things You Can Do to Have a Healthy Baby

2

Notes

_____

_____

_____

_____

_____

_____

_____

_____

_____

_____

_____

_____

Things You Must Not Do

What is it?

Everything you do affects your baby. Some things like smoking, alcohol, and drugs can hurt your baby for life. These things are no-no's during pregnancy.

What do I need to know?

- Start being a mother as soon as you start trying to get pregnant. Stay away from things that can hurt your baby. Here's a list of things that are very bad for your baby:

  - **Smoking or breathing in someone else's smoke**

    Smoking can cause you to lose your baby or have a very small, sick baby. Breathing in someone else's smoke is called second hand smoke. It's very bad for you and your baby.

    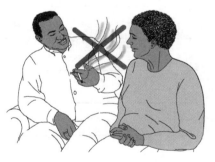

  - **Drinking alcohol**

    Alcohol includes hard liquor, beer, and wine. Alcohol can give your baby birth defects. It can cause mental retardation and other problems for life.

    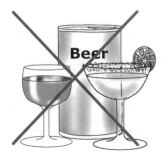

- **Taking street drugs**

  Street drugs like cocaine, speed, crank, and marijuana (pot) can harm your baby's brain. They can also cause your baby to be born too early. Babies of mothers who 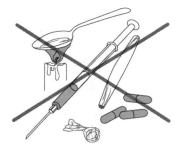 take drugs are often born addicted to drugs. They are born sick and can have problems all their lives.

- **Prescription and over-the-counter medicines**

  Do not take any medicines that you buy at the store. Do not take any medicines ordered by other doctors without talking with 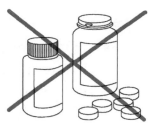 your pregnancy doctor first.

- **Here are other things that can hurt your baby:**

  - Getting x-rays. Tell people you are pregnant when you go for health or dental care.

  - Not getting health care throughout your pregnancy

  - Changing cat litter. You can get an illness that can harm your baby.

  - Touching pet hamsters and guinea pigs. They can carry a disease that can harm your baby.

  - Disease from rats and mice can harm your baby.

  - Eating raw or under cooked meat or fish. You can get an illness that can harm your baby.

- Breathing fumes from cleansers, paint, and other things
- Dieting or not eating healthy food
- Eating or drinking too many things with caffeine in them
- Bad teeth
- Taking hot baths or going into hot tubs

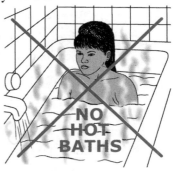

What should I do?

- If you smoke, take drugs, or drink alcohol, stop now. There are support groups and other places that can help you. Ask your doctor for help. You can call the National Drug and Alcohol Treatment hotline at 1-800-662-4357. You can also find a place for help by looking in the front of the phone book under Alcohol and Drug Abuse.

- Stay away from people who smoke. Breathing their smoke is bad for you and your baby.

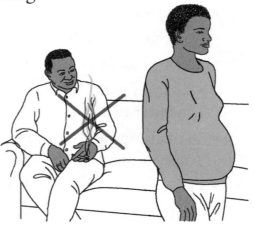

- Go to your doctor. Pregnant women need to see their doctor at least:
  - Once a month in months 1 through 7
  - Every 2 weeks in month 8
  - Every week in month 9
- Your doctor will tell you when to come in.
- Do not take any medicines unless your doctor says it's OK. Ask your doctor for a list of things that are safe to take during pregnancy.
- When you go for health or dental care, tell people that you are pregnant.
- Do not eat or drink too many things that have caffeine in them like coffee, tea, chocolate, and sodas.
- Do these things to protect your baby:
  - If you have a cat, get someone else to change the cat litter.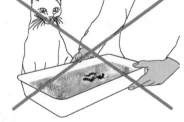
  - Get help if you have rats or mice around your house.
  - Stay away from pet hamsters and guinea pigs. Get others to care for the pet and clean the cage.
  - Always wear gloves if you work in the garden. Wash food from the garden.
  - Do not eat raw meat or fish. Cook your meat well.
  - Do not eat more than 12 ounces of fish a week. Eat fish low in mercury like shrimp, salmon, and canned light tuna. Do not eat fish high in mercury like shark, swordfish, tilefish, king mackerel, or albacore tuna.

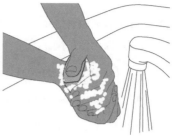

- Wash your hands well with soap and water after touching pets and raw meat.

- Do not take hot baths. Bath water should not be hotter than 100 degrees F. Do not go into hot tubs or steam baths.

- Do not diet during pregnancy. Your baby will not get enough food. This will harm your growing baby.

- Do not skip any meals.

- If you paint a room, open the windows and doors. Avoid using strong cleansers. Stay away from other types of fumes. Fumes can hurt you and your baby.

- See your dentist. Have your teeth fixed.

When do I call my doctor or nurse?

- Call if you want to know if something is safe to do or take during pregnancy.

- Call if you feel very sick and want to know if there is anything you can take.

- Call if you need help to stop smoking, drinking alcohol, or taking drugs.

- You can call the National Drug and Alcohol Treatment hotline at 1-800-662-4357. You can also find a place for help by looking in the front of the phone book under Alcohol and Drug Abuse.

Finding a Doctor or Midwife

What is it?

It means finding a place to go for medical care during your pregnancy.

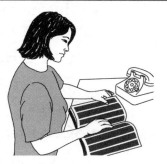

What do I need to know?

- Women need to get medical care throughout pregnancy to have a healthy baby. They need to go to a doctor or nurse midwife soon after they miss their first period.

- The medical care a woman gets when she is pregnant is called prenatal care.

- Pregnant women need to see their doctor or midwife even if they feel well:
  - Once a month during months 1 through 7
  - Every 2 weeks in month 8
  - Every week in month 9

- Your doctor will tell you when to come in.

- If you miss a visit, call right away to set another visit.

- Some women have problems and need to see their doctor more often.

- Medical people work as a team to care for you and your baby while you are pregnant. Here's a list of some of these people:

- **Family Doctor**

  This is a medical doctor who takes care of everyone in the family. Some family doctors have special training to care for pregnant women and deliver babies.

- **Obstetrician-Gynecologist (OB/GYN)**

  This is a medical doctor who specializes in woman's health.

- **Certified Nurse Midwife, or CNM**

  A CNM is a nurse who has special training to care for women during pregnancy. They deliver babies and may assist doctors with C-sections.

- **Physician Assistant, or PA-C**

  A PA-C is a licensed person with special training. PAs work closely with medical doctors when caring for you.

- **Nurse Practitioner, or NP**

  An NP is a nurse with special training to care for you before and after you have your baby.

- **Pediatrician**

  This is a medical doctor who is trained to care for new babies and children.

What should I do?

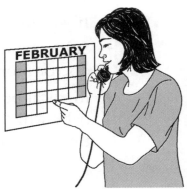

- Call to see a doctor. Do this within 3 weeks of missing your period.
- There are many ways to find a doctor. Here are some things you can do:

- Ask your family doctor where to go for care during your pregnancy.

- If you have a health plan, call the 800 number and ask where to go for health care.

- If you have a friend or family member who is a nurse or works for a doctor, ask them to help you find a doctor.

- Call a hospital in your area for places to go for care during pregnancy.

- Ask a friend who had a baby where she went for health care.

- Ask the doctor or hospital about childbirth education classes.

- Call the health department in your city or county and ask them about clinics and ways to pay.

- Check the front of your phone book under Health Care. Call a clinic like a women's health care clinic.

- Do not miss a doctor's visit because you do not have a ride. If you need a ride, call your health plan or talk to your doctor. They can help you find a ride.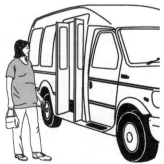

- Go to all your doctor's visits even if you feel well.

When do I call my doctor or nurse?

- Call if you think you may be pregnant.

Special Tests

What is it?

They are tests that tell how your baby is doing.

What do I need to know?

- All women get routine blood and urine (pee) tests while they are pregnant.

- Some women need special tests. Your doctor or nurse will tell you if you need special tests. Here is a list of some special tests:

  ### Ultrasound

  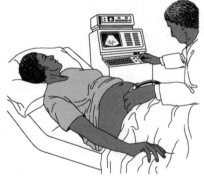

  - Most pregnant women get this test.

  - It is often done in a doctor's office when a woman is 16–20 weeks pregnant.

  - The test uses sound waves to take a picture of your baby. This does not hurt you or baby.

  - It shows how your baby is growing. It tells the doctor about when your baby is due.

  - Jelly is spread on your belly. A device is moved back and forth over your belly.

  - You can see your baby on a TV screen.

Glucose Tolerance Test

- This test checks the amount of sugar in your blood.

- It is done at a lab or in a doctor's office.

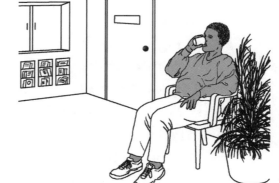

- You will be given a sweet liquid to drink.

- Blood is taken from your arm after you drink the liquid.

The Non-Stress Test

- This test is sometimes done in the later part of pregnancy.

- It is done in a doctor's office or at a hospital.

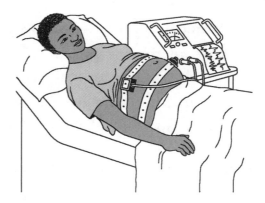

- A device is put on your belly.

- The test checks your baby's heart rate when he moves.

- This test tells if your baby is doing OK.

The Stress Test

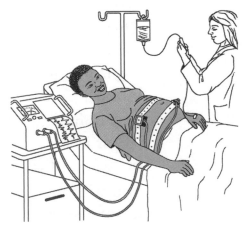

- This test is done at a hospital.
- It checks your baby's heart rate when the uterus gets tight (during contractions).
- A device is put on your belly. It records your baby's heart rate.
- Medicine or other things are used to make your uterus get tight.
- This test checks if your baby will be OK to start labor.

What should I do?

- See a doctor as soon as you think you may be pregnant.
- Your doctor will do the tests you need. He or she will tell you if you need special tests.
- Do what your doctor or nurse tells you. Your doctor will help you have a healthy baby.

When do I call my doctor or nurse?

- Call if you think you may be pregnant.
- Call if you want to know if what you are feeling is normal.
- Call if you have one of the warning signs on pages 11–12.

Eating Right for a Healthy Baby

What is it?

You need to eat healthy food when you are pregnant. You also need to eat a little more than before. Your baby uses the food you eat to grow.

What do I need to know?

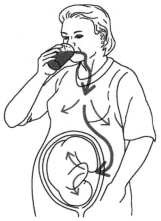

- The food you eat goes to your baby.

- You need to eat healthy food to have a healthy baby. You also need to eat many types of foods. No one food gives your baby all that he or she needs to grow.

- If your weight is normal, plan to gain 25–35 pounds during your pregnancy. You will lose most of the weight after you have your baby.

- The amount of food you need to eat depends on your size and how active you are.

- It's not safe to diet or not eat when you are pregnant. If you do this you can lose or harm your baby for life.

- It's important to eat healthy even when you do not feel like eating. Your baby needs food to grow.

Eating Right for a Healthy Baby

- A pregnant woman needs to eat food every day from each of the 5 food groups. Below is a list of the food groups and the number of servings an average pregnant woman needs to eat.

- Your doctor or nurse will watch your weight and tell you how much you need to eat.

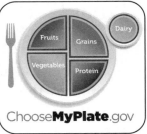

- The website **www.choosemyplate.gov/ pregnancy-breastfeeding.html** can tell you how much food to eat every day.

1. **Meat, Fish, Eggs, and Poultry: Eat 2–3 servings a day.**

   One serving is:

   > 2 eggs or
   >
   > 1 piece of chicken, fish, or lean meat (size of a deck of cards) or
   >
   > 2 tablespoons of peanut butter or
   >
   > ½ cup of cooked beans

   These foods give protein and iron that your baby needs to build a strong, healthy body.

2. **Milk, Yogurt, and Cheese: Eat 3 servings a day.**

   One serving is:

   > 8 ounces of lowfat or nonfat milk or
   >
   > 1 cup lowfat or nonfat yogurt or
   >
   > 2 slices of cheese or
   >
   > ½ cup of lowfat cottage cheese

   These foods give calcium that you and your baby need for strong bones and teeth.

3. **Bread, Cereal, and Pasta: Eat 6 or more servings a day.**

   One serving is:

   > 1 slice of whole grain bread or
   >
   > 1 small roll or muffin or
   >
   > 1 cup dry cereal or
   >
   > ½ cup cooked cereal, rice, or pasta or
   >
   > 8 crackers or
   >
   > One 6-inch tortilla

   These foods give your body energy. Eat whole grain breads and cereals for fiber.

4. **Fruits: Eat 4–5 servings a day.**

   One serving is:

   > 1 medium apple, orange, or banana or
   >
   > ½ grapefruit or
   >
   > ½ cup fresh, frozen, or canned fruit or
   >
   > ¾ cup fruit juice or
   >
   > ¼ cup of raisins

   These foods give you and your baby fiber, vitamin C, and some folic acid.

5. **Vegetables: Eat 5 or more servings a day.**

   One serving is:

   > ½ cup of raw or cooked vegetables or
   >
   > 1 small baked potato or
   >
   > ¾ cup of vegetable juice

These foods give you and your baby fiber, vitamin A, and some folic acid.

- Drink 8–10 glasses of fluids a day.
- There are programs to help pregnant and nursing mothers get the healthy food they need. It's called the WIC (women, infants, and children) program. You can get information about WIC from your doctor's office or by calling WIC. You can find the number for WIC in the front of the phone book under Mother and Infant Health.

What should I do?

- Eat 3 meals and 3 snacks every day.
- Eat healthy food. Here's a sample of healthy eating for 1 day.

Breakfast

6 ounces prune juice

½ cup cooked oatmeal with raisins

1 boiled egg

1 slice of whole wheat toast with 1 teaspoon butter

8 ounces lowfat milk

Morning Snack

1 apple

8 whole wheat crackers

Lunch

1 cup vegetable soup

Ham and cheese
   sandwich with tomato
   and lettuce on whole
   wheat bread

1 banana

8 ounces lowfat milk

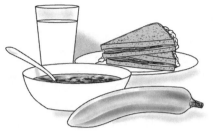

Afternoon Snack

1 cup carrot sticks

1 orange

Dinner

1 cup salad with tomatoes

1–2 tablespoons
   salad dressing

1 small whole grain roll

½ cup brown rice

4 ounces baked chicken

½ cup broccoli

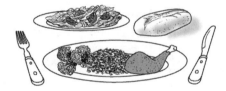

Evening Snack

1 small bran muffin

8 ounces lowfat milk

- Do not eat more than 12 ounces of fish a week. Eat fish low in mercury like shrimp, salmon, or canned light tuna. Avoid fish high in mercury like shark, swordfish, king mackerel, tilefish, or albacore tuna.

Eating Right for a Healthy Baby

- Drink 5–6 glasses of water every day plus 3–4 glasses of milk and other fluids.

- Avoid junk food like sodas, potato chips, and candy. These foods will make you gain too much weight. They won't give your baby what he or she needs to grow.

- If you do not drink milk, ask your doctor what to take to replace the milk.

- Take the vitamin pills that the doctor tells you even if you are eating right.

When do I call my doctor or nurse?

- Call if you are sick to your stomach and you can't keep down any food or fluids for 24 hours.

- Call if you are losing weight.

- Call if you are gaining more than 1 pound a week.

- Call WIC if you need help to buy healthy food. Their phone number is in the front of the phone book under Mother and Infant Health.

Exercise

What is it?

Exercise means being active and moving around.

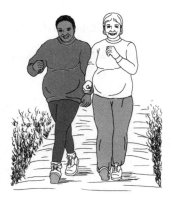

What do I need to know?

- It's safe for most women to be active during pregnancy. Fast walking for 30 minutes every day is good.

- Swimming is good exercise. The water should not feel cold or hot.

- Hot tubs and steam baths are **not good** when you are pregnant.

- Exercise during pregnancy is good. It can:
  - Help you relax.
  - Help back pain and constipation.
  - Reduce swelling in your feet and ankles.
  - Help you get strong for childbirth.

- Women should not start a new sport or a hard exercise program when they are pregnant. A pregnant woman's heart rate should not go over 140 beats per minute.

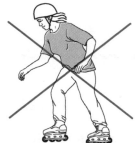

- Pregnant women should not do these things:
  - Do not do things that can lead to falls like horseback riding, downhill skiing, or skating.
  - Do not exercise to the point where you are very tired or out of breath.
  - Do not do sports like soccer where you can get hit in the stomach.
  - Do not exercise in a hot place.
  - Do not let your body get too hot. This can be bad for your baby.
  - Do not exercise flat on your back after the 4th month of pregnancy. This is bad for your blood flow.

What should I do?

- Talk to your doctor about what exercises you can safely do. Ask if there is an exercise class for pregnant women.
- Wear loose clothes. Dress in layers. Take off some layers if you get too hot.
- Wear shoes with good support. Your feet can swell when you are pregnant. You may need a larger shoe size.

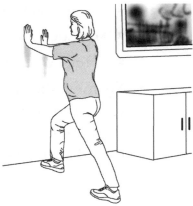

- Start exercising slowly. Do things like stretches and slow walking first. This is called warming up.

- Do not stop exercising all at once. If you are walking fast, walk slowly for the last 10 minutes. This is called cooling down.

- Do not exercise when you are hungry. Eat a light snack 1–2 hours before you exercise.

- Do not hold your breath when you exercise. Breathe in and out.

- You should be able to talk while exercising. If you can't talk, slow down.

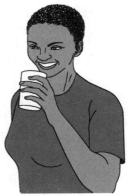

- Drink a glass of water before and after you exercise.

- If your pee is dark, drink more fluids. Dark pee means your body is low on fluids.

- Do these exercises every day in addition to walking or other activities.

Ankle exercise:

This exercise is good for the blood flow in your legs and feet.

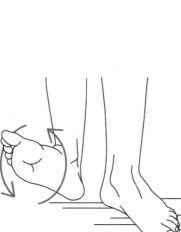

- Sit in a comfortable chair.

- Lift your right foot off the floor.

- Draw a circle in the air with your toes. Do 10 circles.

- Now do 10 circles with the same foot going the other way.
- Put your right foot down. Lift your left foot off the floor.
- Do 10 circles each way with your left foot.
- Do this exercise 2 times a day.

Back exercises:

They are good for a sore back. Do these exercises 2 times a day.

Exercise 1

- Get down on your hands and knees. Keep your neck and head in line with your back.

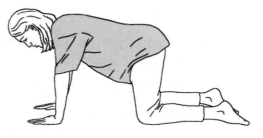

- Hold your back straight. Do not let your back sag.

- Arch your back up like a cat. At the same time roll your head and neck under you.

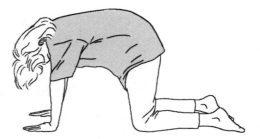

- Tighten your belly and bottom.

- Slowly lower your back flat while lifting your head and neck.

- Do this 10 times.

Exercise 2

- Lie on your right side.
- Hold your left leg below the knee.
- Slowly pull your leg up and out towards your shoulder.

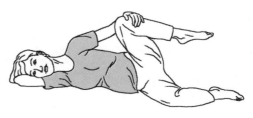

- Hold it while you count to 20.
- Slowly bring your leg down.
- Do this 5 times.
- Turn on your left side. Repeat this 5 times with your right leg.

Stop exercising right away if you get any of these signs:

- You feel weak or dizzy
- You get a headache or you see double
- You have pain anywhere in your body
- You feel your heart racing
- You have trouble breathing
- You start bleeding or leaking fluid from your vagina

When do I call my doctor or nurse?

- Call before you start a new exercise program.
- Call if you want to know if something is safe for you to do.
- Call right away if you have bleeding from the vagina, feel dizzy, or have chest pain.

Expecting a Baby Month by Month

3

Notes

Month 1

What is it?

My baby:

- Baby is called an embryo in the early part of pregnancy.
- Baby's body parts are just starting to form.
- Baby is about a ½ inch long.
- Baby weighs less than 1 ounce.

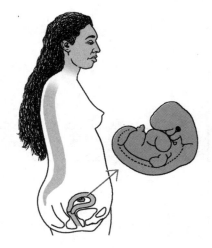

My body:

- You will not have your monthly period while you are pregnant.
- You may feel sick to your stomach. You may throw up a few times a day. This is known as morning sickness.
- Your breasts are sore and may feel bigger.
- You may feel tired.
- You may have gas or heartburn.
- You may need to pee often.
- You may feel the same way you do before you get your period.
- You may feel happy, sad, or moody. You may cry. This is normal. It is called mood swings.

What should I do?

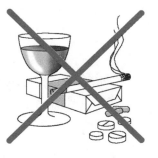

- Do not smoke, drink alcohol, or take street drugs. These things will hurt your baby.

- Do not take any medicines unless your doctor says it's OK. This includes medicines you buy or that another doctor ordered.

- Read about other things you must not do on pages 14–18.

- Eat healthy foods. Read what to eat on pages 25–29.

- Eat foods high in folic acid such as spinach, broccoli, and cereals with added folic acid.

- Do not eat more than 12 ounces of fish a week. Don't eat fish high in mercury like shark, swordfish, tilefish, king mackerel, or albacore tuna.

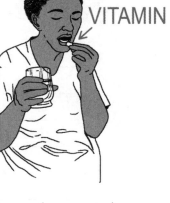

VITAMIN

- It's important to take the vitamins your doctor ordered. If vitamins make your stomach sick, take them after you eat food or at bedtime.

- Try to get a lot of rest.

- Keep your teeth and gums healthy. Brush your teeth with a soft toothbrush. Do this after every meal and at bedtime. Floss your teeth every day. See your dentist for a check-up. Tell the dentist that you are pregnant.

- **Call your doctor or nurse if:**
  - You are very sick to your stomach and can't keep down any fluids or food for 24 hours.
  - You need help to stop smoking, drinking alcohol, or using drugs. You can call 1-800-662-4357 for a place to go for help.
- Go to your doctor. Do this even if you do not feel sick.
- Write down a list of things you want to ask like:
  - I feel happy and sad at the same time. Why do I have so many feelings?
  - I must work to make ends meet. When do I have to stop working?

Questions for my visit on (date) _____:

1. _____

   _____

2. _____

   _____

3. _____

   _____

4. _____

   _____

5. _____

   _____

What will my doctor do?

- You will have a blood or urine (pee) test to check if you are pregnant. This is called a pregnancy test.

- Your doctor will ask you a lot of questions like if you drink alcohol, smoke, or take drugs.

- Tell your doctor the truth. Your doctor is trying to help you have a healthy baby. Your doctor cannot tell other people what you say without your OK. What you say is kept private.

- You will be given a physical exam. This includes checking your heart, lungs, belly, breasts, and legs. The doctor may also check your eyes, ears, and mouth, and feel your neck and breasts for lumps.

- You will have a pelvic exam.

- This exam is done on a table with your legs spread apart. A paper drape will cover you. The doctor will put fingers into your vagina and on your belly. The doctor will feel your cervix and the size, shape, and position of your uterus.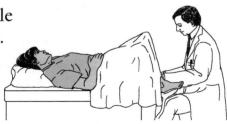

- A special tool called a speculum is put into the vagina to keep it open. Cells are taken from the cervix to test for cancer. This is called a pap smear. This exam does not hurt. Some fluid may be taken from your vagina to test for sexually transmitted diseases, called STDs.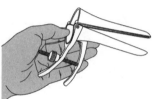

Month 1

- You will have a blood test for sugar and other things.
- You will be asked to have an HIV test. It's important to have this test. A person can have HIV and not know it. HIV can be passed on to a new baby. If you find out early you have HIV, you can take medicine to help you and your baby.
- Your doctor will order prenatal vitamins. Be sure to take your vitamins.
- Talk to your doctor about problems or questions you may have.
- Your doctor will tell you what to do. You may be given things to read. Tell your doctor if you do not understand the information.

Things my doctor told me to do:

_____

_____

_____

_____

_____

_____

_____

_____

_____

Month 2

What is it?

My baby:

- Baby's heart is beating.
- Baby has arms and legs.
- Baby's fingers and toes are forming.
- Baby is about 1 inch long.
- Baby weighs less than 1 ounce.

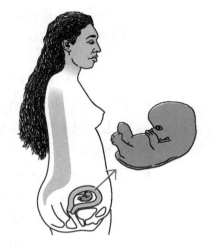

My body:

- You may have gained about 1 or more pounds so far.
- Your breasts may feel bigger and may hurt a little.
- You may throw up every day. This is called morning sickness. It can happen anytime of the day.
- You may feel tired.
- You may need to pee often.
- You may have a hard time having a bowel movement. This is called constipation.
- You may have gas or heartburn.
- You may have headaches.
- You may want to eat a lot of one type of food, like ice cream. This is called a food craving. It's important to eat a healthy diet.

- Your clothes may start feeling tight around the waist.

- This is the time you realize you are going to be a mother. You may think about it a lot. One day you may be happy. Another day you may be worried. These feelings are normal.

What should I do?

- Do not take any medicines unless your doctor says it's OK. This includes medicines you buy or that another doctor ordered.

- Do not smoke, drink alcohol, or use street drugs. If you need help to stop, talk with your doctor or call 1-800-662-4357.

- Stay away from people who smoke. Breathing the smoke is bad for you and your baby.

- Take your vitamins. If they make your stomach sick, try taking them later in the day after you eat food or before you go to sleep.

- If you have morning sickness, read what to do on pages 86–87.

- Read about other things you can do to feel better on pages 88–112.

- Get lots of rest.

- Eat healthy foods. Read what to eat on pages 25–29. Drink at least 8 glasses of fluids a day.

- Read about when to call your doctor on pages 11–12.
- Be sure to see your doctor. Do this even if you feel well.
- Write down a list of things you want to ask, like:
  - I get headaches often. Is this normal?
  - I feel like I have to throw up after lunch. Is this normal?

Questions for my visit on (date) _____:

1. _____

   _____

2. _____

   _____

3. _____

   _____

4. _____

   _____

5. _____

   _____

What will my doctor do?

If this is your first visit to the doctor, see pages 40–42.

- Check your weight and blood pressure.
- Test your urine (pee) for things like sugar and protein.
- Check your hands and feet for swelling.
- Check your legs for veins that may stick out.

- Ask you how you feel.
- Talk about new things you are feeling.
- Tell you what the tests show.

Things my doctor told me to do:

_____

_____

_____

_____

_____

_____

_____

_____

_____

Month 3

What is it?

My baby:

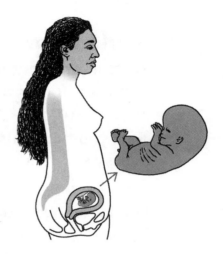

- You can hear your baby's heartbeat.
- Baby's fingers and toes have soft nails.
- Baby is 3–4 inches long.
- Baby weighs almost 1 ounce.

My body:

- You may have gained 2 or more pounds so far. Some women who have bad morning sickness lose a few pounds.
- You may feel many of the same things you felt in month 2.
- Your breasts may be sore.
- You may feel sick to your stomach. You may throw up every day.
- You may feel very tired.
- You may pee often.
- You may be constipated.
- You may have gas or heartburn.

- You may have headaches.
- Your feet may swell.
- Your clothes may feel tight around the waist.

What should I do?

- Read about the warning signs on pages 11–12.
  Call your doctor right away if you think something
  may be wrong.
- Take your vitamins and eat healthy. Drink at least
  8 glasses of fluids a day.
- Get lots of rest.
- Do not smoke, drink alcohol, or take drugs.
  Stay away from people who are smoking.
- Do not take any medicines unless your doctor says it's OK.
- Be sure to see your doctor. Do this even if you feel good.
- Write down a list of things you want to ask, like:
  - I'm so tired all the time. Is this normal?
    When will I feel better?
  - When will I know the sex of my baby?

Questions for my visit on (date) _____:

1. _____

   _____

2. _____

   _____

3. _____

_____

4. _____

_____

5. _____

_____

What will my doctor do?

If this is your first visit to the doctor, see pages 40–42.

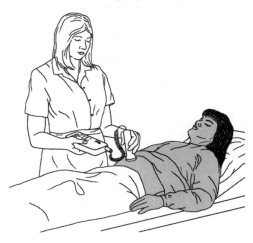

- Check your weight and blood pressure.

- Check baby's heartbeat. This is done using a special device put on your belly.

- May test your urine (pee) for protein and sugar. If there is sugar, other tests may be done.

- Check your hands and feet for swelling.

- Check your legs for veins that may stick out.

- Your doctor may do an ultrasound. Read about this test on page 22.

Things my doctor told me to do:

_____

_____

_____

_____

_____

_____

_____

_____

_____

_____

Month 4

What is it?

My baby:

- Baby can hear your voice.
- Baby moves and kicks. You may or may not feel the baby moving.
- Baby begins to suck and swallow.
- Baby is 5–7 inches long.
- Baby weighs about 6 ounces.

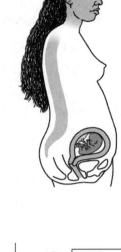

My body:

- You have gained about 3–4 pounds so far.
- Your breasts are getting bigger.
- You may feel better and have more energy.
- Morning sickness may be gone.

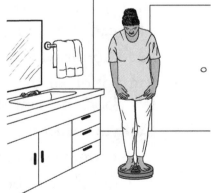

- You may feel like eating more.
- You may pee less often.
- You may still be constipated.
- You may have a small amount of white vaginal discharge.

- You may have gas or heartburn.
- You may have some headaches.
- Your gums may bleed. Use a soft toothbrush and floss. Go to a dentist for a check up.
- Your ankles, feet, and hands may swell a little.
- Your belly is getting bigger. You start to look pregnant.
- This may be the time you start telling people you are going to have a baby.

What should I do?

- Take the vitamins your doctor ordered every day. Do not take any other medicines without checking with your doctor first.
- Eat healthy meals and snacks. Read what foods to eat on pages 25–29.
- Do not wear clothes that are tight around your belly. This can give you an upset stomach.
- Read about what to do for heartburn on pages 88–89.
- Rub lotion or oil on your belly every day. It's good for your skin.
- **Call your doctor or nurse if you have any of these signs:**
  - Bleeding or watery fluid from the vagina
  - Pains in your belly
  - You feel very thirsty
  - Headaches or blurred vision
  - Fever or chills
  - Other warning signs (see pages 11–12)

- Visit your doctor even if you feel well.
- Write down a list of things you want to ask, like:
  - Where will I have my baby?
  - I have bad burning in my stomach. Is there something I can take?
  - I work all day. By noon my feet are swollen and my shoes are tight. Is this normal?

Questions for my visit on (date) _____:

1. _____

   _____

2. _____

   _____

3. _____

   _____

4. _____

   _____

5. _____

   _____

What will my doctor do?

- Your doctor will tell you about a screening blood test for your baby.
- Do a blood test.
- Check your weight and blood pressure.

- Check baby's size and how big your uterus is. This is done by feeling the outside of your belly.
- Check baby's heartbeat.
- May test your urine (pee) for protein and sugar. If there is sugar, other tests may be done.
- Check your hands and feet for swelling.
- Check your legs for veins that may stick out.
- Talk about how you are feeling and what the tests show.

Things my doctor told me to do:

_____

_____

_____

_____

_____

_____

_____

_____

_____

Month 5

What is it?

My baby:

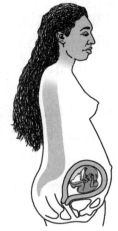

- Baby kicks and moves a lot.
- Baby has hair and fingernails.
- Baby's skin starts to be covered with a white cheesy coat.
- Baby sleeps and wakes up many times a day.
- Baby may get hiccups.
- Baby starts to make sucking motions.
- Baby grows as much as 2 inches this month. Baby is about 10–12 inches long.
- Baby weighs ½–1 pound.

My body:

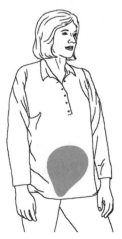

- You have gained about 8 pounds so far in the pregnancy.
- The top of the uterus is near your belly button.
- You feel your baby moving almost every day. Baby has lots of room in your belly. It may feel like butterflies or gas at first.

- You may feel some dull aches in your lower belly. This is because your belly is getting bigger.

- You may feel your heart beating faster.

- You are starting to get a dark line down the center of your belly. You may have dark spots on your face. These skin changes are normal. They often go away after you have your baby.

- Your breasts are a lot bigger. Your nipples are getting darker in color. Your breasts may leak clear, sticky fluid. This is early breast milk. It is called colostrum. It is normal.

- You may have more white discharge from your vagina.

- Your back may hurt.

- You are always hungry. You may want to eat a lot of sweets.

What should I do?

- Keep lots of healthy food around for snacks, like:
  - Carrot and celery sticks
  - Fruits like bananas and apples
  - Yogurt
  - Peanut butter and whole grain crackers

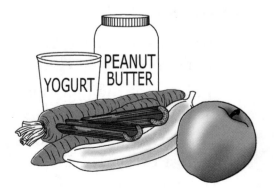

- Keep your face out of the sun. The sun will make the spots on your face darker. Use sunscreen with an SPF of at least 20. Wear a hat to keep the sun off your face.

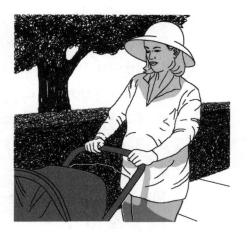

- Wear good walking shoes with flat heels. Try not to stand for a long time.

- Wear a bra with good support. This will help your breasts feel less sore. You can buy a good bra at a store that sells clothes for pregnant women.

- Read about early labor on pages 118–121. Call your doctor right away if you have any signs.

- Read about other warning signs on pages 11–12.

- Rub lotion or oil on your belly every day.

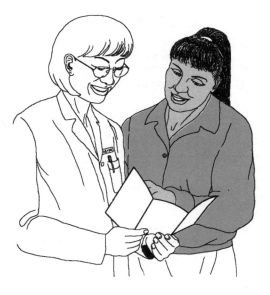

- Ask your doctor about classes to get ready for childbirth.

- Talk with your doctor about what birth control you will use after you have your baby.

- Ask your partner or a friend or family member to be your labor partner or coach. This person will:
  - Go to childbirth classes with you
  - Take you to the hospital if possible
  - Comfort you during labor
  - Time your contractions
  - Remind you how to breathe during labor
- Plan how you will get to the hospital.
- Be sure to see your doctor. Do this even if you feel well.
- Write down a list of things you want to ask, like:
  - I have itching around the vagina. What can I use to take away the itch?
  - My pee is darker in color. Is something wrong?

Questions for my visit on (date) _____:

1. _____

   _____

2. _____

   _____

3. _____

   _____

4. _____

   _____

5. _____

   _____

What will my doctor do?

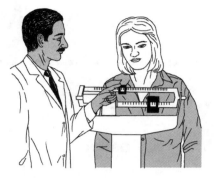

- Check your weight and blood pressure.
- Check baby's size and how big your uterus is.
- May test your urine (pee).
- Check baby's heartbeat.
- You may have an ultrasound. This test checks how baby is growing. Turn to page 22 to read about this test.
- Your doctor will tell you how things look, and answer your questions. He or she may tell you some things to do.

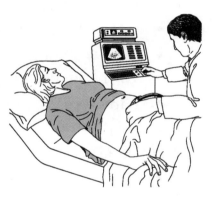

Things my doctor told me to do:

_____

_____

_____

_____

_____

_____

_____

Month 6

What is it?

My baby:

- Baby kicks and moves a lot.
- Baby starts to open the eyes.
- Baby's lungs are forming.
- Baby is about 12–14 inches long.
- Baby weighs about 1½ pounds.

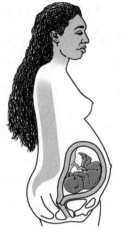

My body:

- You have gained about 10–12 pounds so far.
- Your belly is getting bigger. The skin itches.
- Your uterus is as big as a soccer ball. The top of your uterus is about 2 inches above your belly button.
- Your shoes may feel tight. Your face may look puffy. This happens because your body is holding in water.
- You may get cramps in your legs and feet at night.
- You may have hemorrhoids (HEM-ma-roidz). These are swelling of the veins in your rectum. They can bleed. Tell your doctor or nurse.
- Your nose may feel stuffy.

Month 6

What should I do?

- Try not to scratch the skin on your belly. Rub lotion or oil on your belly every day.

- Read about early labor on pages 118–121. Know what to do if you get any signs.

- Read about what to do for hemorrhoids on pages 99–100.

- Read about swelling of the feet on pages 104–107.

- **Call your doctor or nurse if you have any of these signs:**

  - The uterus gets tight (feels hard). This happens every 10–15 minutes or more often and does not improve with resting. This is called having contractions.

  - Cramps in your belly as if you are starting your period.

  - You have an itchy rash on your belly.

  - Dull lower back pain. It is not the same as your normal backache.

  - Pressure in your pelvis that feels like the baby is pushing down.

  - Thick vaginal discharge with some blood.

  - Fluid leaking or gushing from your vagina.

  - You feel faint or dizzy.

  - Bad headaches or your vision is blurred.

  - A feeling that something is not right.

- It is very important to see your doctor. Do this even if you feel well.
- Write down a list of things you want to ask, like:
  - I get short of breath when I do housework. Is this OK?
  - My nose is stuffy. What can I do to breathe easier?
  - I get bad leg cramps at night. What can I do?

Questions for my visit on (date) _____:

1. _____

    _____

2. _____

    _____

3. _____

    _____

4. _____

    _____

5. _____

    _____

What will my doctor do?

- Check your weight and blood pressure.
- May test your urine (pee).
- Listen to baby's heartbeat.

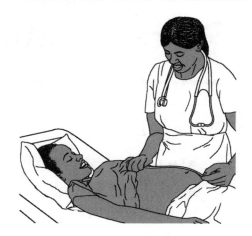

- Feel and measure the outside of your belly. This tells how big your baby is.
- Look at your hands, feet, and ankles for swelling.
- Talk to you about problems you may have.
- Answer your questions.
- Tell you some things to do.

Things my doctor told me to do:

_____

_____

_____

_____

_____

_____

_____

_____

_____

Month 7

What is it?

My baby:

- Baby kicks and stretches for exercise.
- Baby sucks its thumb.
- Baby is about 15 inches long.
- Baby weighs about 3 pounds.

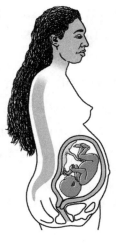

My body:

- You have gained about 16–20 pounds by now. You will gain 1 pound a week during this month.
- You may start getting stretch marks on your belly and breasts.
- Your breasts are sore. They may leak clear, sticky fluid.
- You may feel tired. This is normal. You may have trouble sleeping.
- You feel life inside you. Your baby moves often. The kicking feels stronger.
- You may have more white discharge from your vagina.
- Your gums may bleed when you brush your teeth.

- You may feel hot all the time. This is normal. You may sweat a lot. Sweating cools you. It also makes you lose body fluids. That's why you need to drink a lot of fluids.

- You may have more swelling in your feet and ankles.

- You may start to feel your uterus get tight and then relax. This is called having contractions.

- You may feel unsteady when you walk. This is normal because your belly sticks out.

- You need to pee often. This is normal because your baby is pressing on your bladder.

- You may have an upset stomach (heartburn) after eating. Your stomach is being squeezed by your baby.

What should I do?

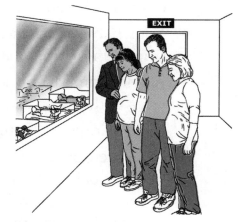

- Go to childbirth classes. They will help you to get ready for labor. Bring your labor partner.

- Take a tour of the hospital where you will deliver.

- Read about early labor on pages 118–121.

- **Call your doctor or nurse right away if you have any of these signs:**

  - Your uterus starts to tighten (feels hard). This happens every 10–15 minutes, or more often, and does not get better with rest. This is called having contractions. Contractions make the cervix open so the baby can pass.

- Cramps in your belly as if you are starting your period.
- Dull lower back pain. It is not the same as your normal backache.
- Pressure in your pelvis that feels like the baby is pushing down.
- Thick vaginal discharge with some blood.
- Fluid leaking or gushing from your vagina.

- Do not rub or pull your nipples to get them ready for breastfeeding. This can start early labor. People may tell you to do this but you do not need to do it.

- A healthy baby kicks, moves, and twists many times a day. Count how often your baby moves. Do this every day. This is called kick counts.

- Your baby is most active after you eat or drink something cold or after you walk for 5–10 minutes.

- A good time to do kick counts is after a meal or after your bedtime snack. Here is what you do:

  - Lie down on your left side.
  - Write down the time you feel your baby's 1st move. It can be a kick, roll, or twist. Use the chart on page 70.
  - Write a check mark (✓) for each time your baby moves.
  - Write down the time you feel the 5th move.
  - Ask your doctor how often you should feel your baby move.

- Fill in the chart on page 70 every day. It will help you keep track of how often your baby moves. Show it to your doctor.

- Call your doctor right away if your baby moves less than 5 times in 1 hour or you do not feel baby move.

- There are other ways to keep track of how often your baby moves. Talk to your doctor about what you should do.

- If you have burning in your stomach, try eating 5 or 6 smaller meals a day. Do not lie down after eating. Read about other things to do for heartburn on pages 88–89.

- Wear flat walking shoes. Be careful not to fall. Read how to stay safe on pages 114–117.

- Sit with your legs up or lie down a few times a day.

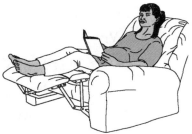

- Do not add salt to your food. Avoid foods that have a lot of salt. Salt makes your body hold water. This will give you more swelling. Read about other things to do for swelling of the feet on pages 104–107.

- Brush your teeth with a soft toothbrush. Do this after every meal and at bedtime. Floss your teeth every day. See the dentist for a check-up. Tell the dentist that you are pregnant.

- Be sure to drink 8–10 glasses of fluids every day. Avoid fruit juices with added sugar. They can give you high blood sugar and too much weight gain.

- Bathe more often if you feel hot. Dress in layers so you can take clothes off if you get too hot.

- Wear a bra that fits well and gives you good support.

- Pee when you feel the need. Do not try to hold your urine (pee). Do Kegel exercises (see page 102).

- Do not push your stomach out when you stand or walk. Do the exercises for your back on pages 93–94.

- Be sure to get enough rest. Sleep on your side with a pillow between your legs and under your belly.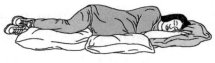

- Read what to do if you have trouble sleeping on pages 111–112.

- Be sure to see your doctor. Do this even if you do not feel sick.

- Write down a list of things you want to ask, like:

  - Is it still OK to have sex?

  - I have bad constipation and hemorrhoids. Is there something I can take?

  - How do I find a doctor for my baby?

Questions for my visit on (date) _____:

1. _____

   _____

2. _____

   _____

3. _____

   _____

4. _____

_____

5. _____

_____

What will my doctor do?

- Check your weight and blood pressure.
- May test your urine (pee).
- Do blood tests.
- Listen to baby's heartbeat.
- Feel and measure the outside of your belly. This tells how big your baby is.
- Look at your hands, feet, and ankles for swelling.
- Talk to you about problems you may have.
- Answer your questions.
- Tell you some things to do.
- Order other special tests.

Things my doctor told me to do:

_____

_____

_____

_____

_____

_____

Kick Counts in Month 7

Date	Time 1st kick	Put a ✓ for each kick	Time 5th kick
Sample	8:30 pm	✓ ✓ ✓ ✓ ✓	9:35 pm

Month 8

What is it?

My baby:

- Baby is getting too big to move around but still kicks and rolls.
- Baby is about 18 inches long.
- Baby weighs about 5 pounds.

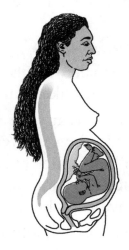

My body:

- You have gained 20–24 pounds so far.
- You may feel like you are running out of space in your belly. Your uterus is about 4 inches above your belly button.
- Your pelvic joints hurt. This is normal. Your joints are starting to relax for delivery.
- Hemorrhoids may be a big problem. Baby's head is pushing down. This causes swelling of the veins in your rectum.
- You may have more stomach upset and gas.
- You may feel stronger contractions in your uterus.
- You may feel you are not getting enough air. This is normal. The top of your uterus is right under your ribs.

- You may be clumsy when you walk.
- You may pee when you laugh or cough. This is normal, but tell your doctor. Be sure it is pee and not other fluid leaking.

What should I do?

- Eat smaller meals more often. Avoid eating foods that make gas like beans.

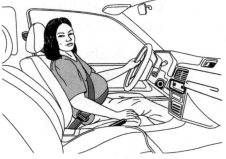

- Always wear your seat belt in the car. Wear the lap belt under your belly. Place the shoulder belt above your belly.
- If you go on a long trip, stop every hour. Get out of the car and walk around for 5 minutes.
- Wear flat walking shoes. Do not try to hurry or run. You can fall because you are carrying an extra 15–20 pounds in front of you.
- Be very careful not to fall in the shower or the tub. Read about other things to do to stay safe on pages 114–117.
- Do not rub or pull your nipples to get them ready for breastfeeding. This can start early labor. People may tell you to do this, but do not do it.
- Pee when you feel the need. Do Kegel exercises (see page 102). It's good for the muscles that hold urine (pee). Strong muscles will also help you during labor.

- Count every day how often your baby kicks or moves (see page 66). Write down your kick counts on the chart on page 76. Call your doctor right away if your baby does not move or moves less often.

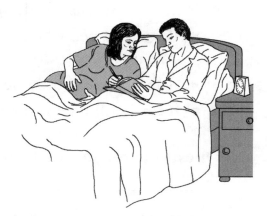

- **Call your doctor or go to the hospital if you have any of these signs:**

  - More than 4 contractions an hour
  - Pain or pressure with contractions
  - Bright red blood from your vagina
  - Gush of fluid leaking from your vagina
  - Sudden weight gain. More swelling of your feet, ankles, face, and hands
  - Bad headaches
  - You see double or things look blurred
  - Pain or burning when you pee
  - Heat, pain, or redness in one or both legs

- In the 8th month your doctor will want to see you every 2 weeks. Go to all your visits. Do this even if you feel fine.

- Write down a list of things you want to ask, like:
  - I start to pee when I sneeze or cough. What should I do?
  - I feel dizzy sometimes. Is this normal?
  - Can I still take tub baths?

Questions for my visit on (date) _____:

1. _____
   _____
2. _____
   _____
3. _____
   _____
4. _____
   _____
5. _____
   _____

What will my doctor do?

- Check your weight and blood pressure.
- May test your urine (pee).
- Your doctor may do more blood tests.
- Listen to baby's heartbeat.
- Feel and measure the outside of your belly. This tells how big your baby is.

Month 8

- Look at your hands, feet, and ankles for swelling.
- Talk to you about problems you may have.
- Answer your questions.
- Tell you some things to do.

Things my doctor told me to do:

_____

_____

_____

_____

_____

_____

_____

_____

_____

Kick Counts in Month 8

Date	Time 1st kick	Put a ✓ for each kick	Time 5th kick
Sample	8:30 pm	✓ ✓ ✓ ✓ ✓	9:35 pm

Month 9

What is it?

My baby:

- Baby has little space to move.

- The lungs and other parts of the body are formed.

- Baby drops during this month. This means baby's head moves down into your pelvis.

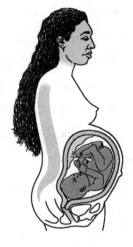

- Baby is about 20 inches long.

- Baby gains about a ½ pound a week. By the end of the 9th month, baby weighs between 6 and 9 pounds.

Your body:

- You may gain very little weight this month. You may not feel like eating.

- Your body is starting to get ready for labor. Here are some changes you may have:

    - Contractions come more often.

    - There's more vaginal discharge. It has pink and brown streaks.

    - Your cervix is starting to open and thin out.

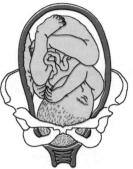

- The mucous plug in the cervix comes out. You will see a pink-brown vaginal discharge. This is called the bloody show.
- The baby drops down in your belly.

- Your breathing is easier after baby drops.
- You will need to pee often after baby drops. Baby is pressing on your bladder.
- Your belly button may stick out.
- You may have some large veins in your legs.
- You may have more swelling of the feet and ankles.
- You may feel tired.
- You may have a lot of trouble sleeping. This is normal.

What should I do?

- A healthy baby moves many times a day. Your baby is most active after you eat or drink something cold or go for a walk. Count how often your baby moves every day. Write the number of times your baby moves on the chart on page 83. Show the chart to your doctor.
- Rest as much as you can.
- Eat healthy food. Do this even if you do not feel hungry.
- Read what to do for large veins in your legs on pages 110–111.
- Read what to do for swollen feet on pages 104–107.

- Make sure you have a ride to the hospital.

- Know how to find your labor partner during the day and at night.

- Know what you will be using for birth control after your baby is born.

- Count how often your contractions come and how long they last. Here is what you do:

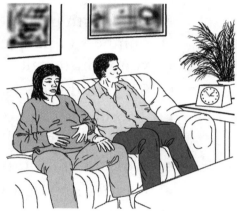

  - Put your hands on your belly.

  - Feel your belly get hard.

  - Count how many seconds it takes for your belly to get soft. That's how long the contraction lasted.

  - The number of minutes it takes for your belly to get hard again is how far apart your contractions are.

- **Call your doctor right away or go to the hospital if you have any of these signs:**

  - Your baby moves less or not at all

  - Bleeding from the vagina

  - Gush or slow leak of fluid from the vagina

  - Green colored fluid from your vagina

  - Your vision is blurred or you see spots

  - You feel very dizzy or faint.

  - You have constant or very bad headaches.

- Pack a bag of things to take to the hospital, like: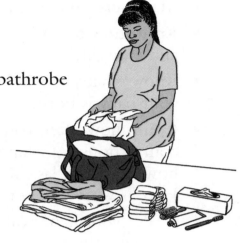
  - Camera
  - A nightgown and/or bathrobe
  - Book to read
  - Book with phone numbers of people you want to call
  - Socks and slippers
  - Toothbrush and other personal things
  - Nursing bra and pads
  - Clothes for you to wear home
  - Clothes for your baby
  - Baby blanket
  - Car seat
- Your doctor will want to see you every week during the last month. Be sure to go to all your visits. Tell your doctor about new things you are feeling.
- Write down a list of things you want to ask, like:
  - How will I know when labor starts?
  - What should I do when labor starts?
  - Baby's movements feel different. Is everything OK?

Questions for my visit on (date) _____:

1. _____

   _____

2. _____

   _____

3. _____

   _____

4. _____

   _____

5. _____

   _____

What will my doctor do?

- Your doctor may do a stress or non-stress test. Read about these tests on pages 23–24.
- Check your weight and blood pressure.
- May test your urine (pee).
- Check baby's heartbeat.
- Check you for signs of problems.
- Talk to you about new things you may be feeling.
- Your doctor may do a pelvic exam to feel your cervix around week 38–40. This may tell if your cervix is ready for labor or has started opening.

Month 9

Things my doctor told me to do:

_____

_____

_____

_____

_____

_____

_____

_____

_____

_____

Kick Counts in Month 9

Date	Time 1st kick	Put a ✔ for each kick	Time 5th kick
Sample	8:30 pm	✓ ✓ ✓ ✓ ✓	9:35 pm

Some Discomforts You May Have

4

Notes

Sick Stomach and Throwing Up (Morning Sickness)

What is it?

It is feeling sick to your stomach (nausea) with or without throwing up (vomiting). It is also known as morning sickness. It can happen anytime of the day. It is often worse in the morning.

What do I need to know?

- About half of all pregnant women have morning sickness. It often goes away by the 4th month.
- It can be the first sign of pregnancy.
- Morning sickness is worse when the stomach is empty.
- The smell of food can make you want to throw up.
- Foods that you used to like may not smell or taste good to you.

What should I do?

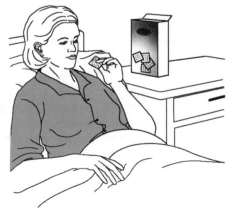

- Keep plain unsalted crackers or rice cakes by your bed. Eat some crackers before you get out of bed in the morning.
- Get out of bed slowly.

Sick Stomach and Throwing Up

- Do not eat or smell foods that make you feel sick.
- Do not let your stomach get empty. It's normal to eat 5 or 6 smaller meals a day when you are pregnant.
- Do not drink fluids with meals. Drink fluids between meals.
- Carry food with you for snacks when you go out.
- Eat a snack before you go to bed at night, like a bran muffin and milk.
- These foods are easier to keep down on a sick stomach:
  - Unsalted crackers
  - Hard boiled eggs
  - Plain popcorn (no butter)
  - Plain baked potatoes
  - Dry cereal
  - Dry toast
  - Rice cakes

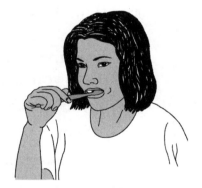

- Do not take any medicines unless your doctor tells you.
- Brush your teeth after you throw up.

When do I call my doctor or nurse?

- Call if you have pain in your belly.
- Call if you can't keep down any food or fluids for 24 hours.
- Call if you are losing weight.

Burning in Your Stomach (Heartburn)

What is it?

It is a burning feeling in your upper stomach and chest. It's also known as heartburn.

What do I need to know?

- Many women get heartburn. It has nothing to do with the heart.

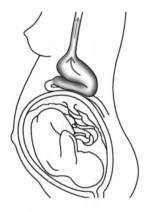

- The muscles of the stomach relax during pregnancy. The growing baby presses on the stomach. This causes food and fluid from the stomach to back up. This gives you a burning feeling in your chest.

- These things can give you heartburn or make it worse:
  - Coffee, tea, chocolate, and cola drinks
  - Spicy and greasy foods
  - Lying down after a meal
  - Eating a large meal

What should I do?

- Eat 5 or 6 smaller meals a day.
- Drink fluids between meals, not with meals.

Burning in Your Stomach (Heartburn)

- Avoid spicy and greasy foods.
- Do not eat or drink foods with caffeine, like coffee and chocolate.
- Avoid lying down for 1 hour after a meal.
- Do not wear clothes that are tight around your belly.
- Do not lie flat. Keep your head and shoulders up about 8 inches. Put something under your mattress to raise the top.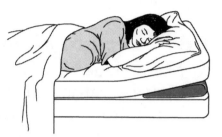
- Eat yogurt or cottage cheese or drink milk when you have heartburn.
- If you have bad heartburn, ask your doctor if you can take antacids.

When do I call my doctor or nurse?
- Call if you tried the things listed above and you still have bad heartburn.

Backache

What is it?

It is pain in your back.

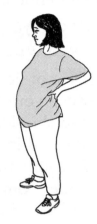

What do I need to know?

- Many women have back pain during pregnancy. The extra weight from the growing baby puts pressure on your back.

- Pregnant women often push their stomach out when they stand or walk. This strains the back.

- Pregnant women who have good posture have less back pain.

- Some women get pain down their leg. It comes from the baby pressing on a nerve in the back. Lying on the other side can take the pressure off the nerve.

- Back pain can be a sign of early labor.

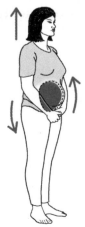

What should I do?

- Do not push your stomach out when you stand or walk. Keep your back straight. Tuck your bottom under.

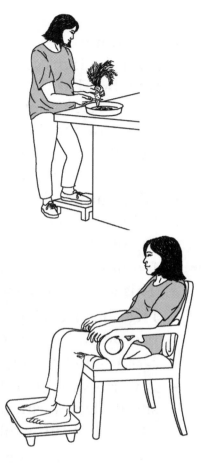

- Try not to stand for more than 30 minutes. If you must stand for a long time, put one foot on a low stool. Change feet every 10–15 minutes. Walk around every 30–40 minutes.

- Wear flat shoes with good support.

- Sit in a chair with good back and arm support. Use a small pillow to support your lower back. Put your feet up on a stool. This takes the pressure off your back.

- Do not sit in one place for longer than 1 hour. Get up and move around every 30–40 minutes.

- Try to lie down on your side a few times a day. Put a pillow between your legs and under your stomach. This rests your back.

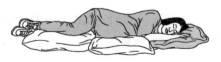

- Try to get someone to help you do work around the house.

Backache

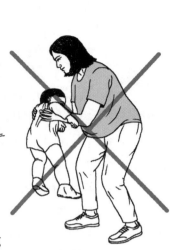

- If you must lift, do it the right way. Bend at the knees. Keep your back straight. Lift with your arms and legs.

- When lifting, hold things close to your body.

- Do not lift heavy things. This can strain your back.

- Heat helps back pain. Put a heating pad on your back for 20 minutes 2 or 3 times a day. Use the low setting. Wrap the heating pad in a towel.

- A warm shower or bath will relax your back. The water should feel warm, not hot. Do not take hot baths or sit in a hot tub while you are pregnant.

- Ask someone to give you a back rub.

- Tylenol is the only medicine that you can take that may help back pain.

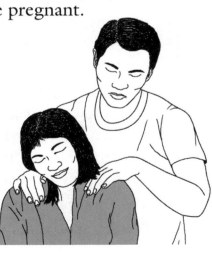

- When getting out of bed, turn on your side and push yourself up with your arms, keeping your back straight.

- Here are a few exercises you can do to help your back.

Exercise 1

- Get down on your hands and knees. Keep your neck and head in line with your back.

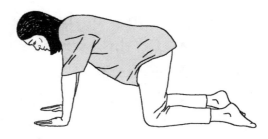

- Hold your back straight. Do not let your back sag.

- Arch your back like a cat. At the same time tuck your head and neck down.

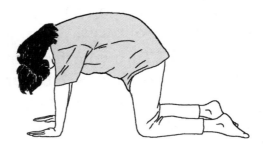

- Slowly lower your back flat while lifting your head and neck.

- Repeat this 10 times.

- Do this exercise 2 times a day.

Exercise 2

- Lie on your right side.

- Hold your left leg below the knee.

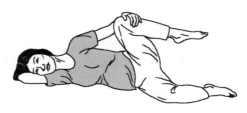

- Slowly pull your leg up and out towards your shoulder.

- Hold it while you count to 20.

- Slowly bring your leg down.
- Do this 5 times.
- Turn on your left side. Repeat this 5 times with your right leg.
- Do this exercise 2 times a day.

Exercise 3

- Hold on to a chair.
- Keep your back straight.
- Lower your body by bending and opening your legs.
- Turn your feet out slightly. Keep your feet flat on the floor.
- Count to 20, then slowly stand up.
- Repeat this 4 more times.
- Do this exercise 2 times a day.

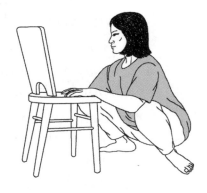

When do I call my doctor or nurse?

- Call if you did the things above, but you still have a lot of pain in your back.
- Call if the pain is not the same as your normal backache.
- Call if you have cramps that feel like you are going to have your period.
- Call if you have signs of early labor on pages 118–119.

Constipation

What is it?

It is hard, dry bowel movements (BMs) that are hard to push out.

What do I need to know?

- Most pregnant women have some constipation.
  - The growing uterus presses on the bowels and slows them.
  - Iron in vitamins can make you constipated. Do not stop taking your vitamins.
- Some things can make you **more** constipated:
  - Not drinking 8–10 glasses of fluids
  - Not being active
  - Not enough fiber in your diet
  - Not going to the bathroom when you first feel the urge
  - Eating a lot of rice and pasta
- Pregnant women should not take medicine (laxatives) to help them have BMs.
- Straining for a bowel movement can make hemorrhoids worse.

- Passing large, hard BMs can cause sores in the end of the rectum (anus). They are very painful. They often bleed.
- Drinking warm water with some lemon can help you have a BM.

What should I do?

- The best thing you can do is eat foods high in fiber, like:

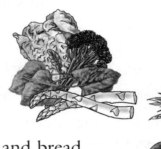

  - Fresh fruits and vegetables
  - Whole grain cereal and bread
  - Dried fruit like prunes, apricots, and raisins
  - Bran

- Drink warm or hot fluids when you wake up. Eat breakfast every day.

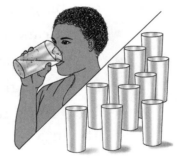

- Drink 8–10 glasses of fluids a day. Prune juice is good for constipation.

- Be active every day. Walk at least 30 minutes a day.

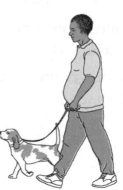

- Do not take any medicines (laxatives). Talk to your doctor if constipation is bad. A stool softener like Colace may be ordered by your doctor.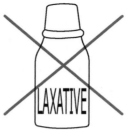

- Try not to strain for a bowel movement. Straining will make hemorrhoids worse.

- Do not ignore the urge to have a BM. Go as soon as you feel the urge.

- You can train your bowels to move at the same time every day. Here is what you can do:

  - Set a time each day to go. After breakfast is a good time.

  - You do not need to wait until you feel the urge to go.

  - Sit on the toilet for 5–10 minutes. Your body will empty itself if you relax.

  - Try drinking a glass of warm water.

  - Do not strain.

  - Do not sit for longer than 10 minutes.

  - If you do not go, try again 20 or 30 minutes after your next meal.

- If your constipation is very bad, try adding wheat bran to food. You can buy it at the food store. It has no taste.

  - It can give you gas, so start with only ½–1 teaspoon.

  - Mix it into applesauce or prune juice.

- Drink a full glass of water after taking the bran.
- You can also put bran on cereal or mix it in cooked foods.
- Do not use more than 2 tablespoons of bran a day.

When do I call my doctor or nurse?

- Call if you tried the things above, but you are still constipated.
- Call if you have not had a bowel movement in more than 3 days.
- Call if you have pains in your belly.

Hemorrhoids

What is it?

Hemorrhoids (HEM-ma-roidz) are swollen veins in and around the rectum.

What do I need to know?

- Many women get hemorrhoids during pregnancy.
- You can get hemorrhoids inside and outside the rectum.
- Hemorrhoids come from the baby pressing on the rectal veins.
- Hemorrhoids can cause itching, pain, and bleeding. Bleeding from hemorrhoids is not a sign of a problem with the pregnancy.
- Constipation makes hemorrhoids worse.
- There are things you can do to help hemorrhoids.
- Hemorrhoids often go away after you have your baby.

What should I do?

- Read how to prevent constipation on pages 95–98.
- Keep pressure off the rectal veins by doing these things:
    - Lie down on your side a few times a day, if you can. Do this when you are reading or watching TV.

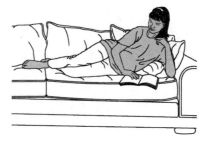

- Sleep on your side, not on your back.
- Do not sit or stand for a long time.
- Do not strain when you have a BM.

- Keep your rectal area clean. Wash it with soap and water after having a BM.

- Put ice packs on your hemorrhoids 2 or 3 times a day.

- Ask your doctor if you can use over-the-counter medicines like Preparation H or glycerin suppositories.

- Do Kegel exercises (see page 102). It helps the blood flow in the area.

- Sitting in warm water helps hemorrhoids. This is called a sitz bath. Here is what you do:

  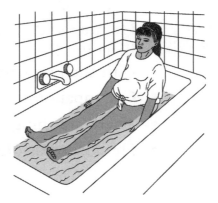

  - Sit in warm water in the tub for 20 minutes 2 or 3 times a day.
  - The water can be a little warmer than your usual bath water.
  - The water should not cover your belly. It's only for your bottom.

- Sit on an ice pack after the sitz bath. The cold will help shrink the hemorrhoids.

When do I call my doctor or nurse?

- Call if you have a lot of pain from hemorrhoids.
- Call if you are afraid to have a BM because of hemorrhoid pain.

You Need to Pee Often

What is it?

You need to pee more often than before you were pregnant.

What do I need to know?

- Most women pee more often when they are pregnant. This is normal.
  - The growing uterus presses on the bladder.
  - Your body makes more pee when you are pregnant.
- It's important to drink 8–10 glasses of fluids a day.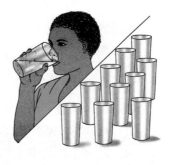
- Some pregnant women get a bladder or kidney infection. This is bad. It can cause early labor. The signs of an infection are:
  - Needing to pee often but going only small amounts.
  - Pain or burning when you pee.
  - Blood in the urine.
  - Chills or fever.
  - Pain in your back or belly.
- Later in pregnancy, some women pee when they laugh or cough. This is normal.

What should I do?

- Pee when you feel the urge. Do not try to hold it in. This can cause an infection.

- Try to empty your bladder all the way, but do not strain.

- Drink 8–10 glasses of fluids every day. To avoid getting up too many times at night, drink your fluids before 5 p.m.

- Avoid drinking coffee, tea, and sodas.

- Do Kegel exercises (see below) to make the muscles around your vagina strong. This will help you hold your urine (pee).

- Here is how to do a Kegel exercise:
    - Squeeze your muscles as if you are stopping pee from coming out.
    - Hold it tight and count to 6. Do not hold your breath.
    - Slowly relax the muscles.
    - This counts as doing the exercise 1 time.
    - Squeeze and relax the muscle 10 times. Do this exercise 5 times a day.

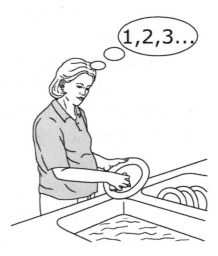

- You can do Kegel exercises anywhere. You can do them while watching TV, reading a book, or washing dishes.

- Make Kegel exercises part of your daily routine.
  - Do a set of 10 while brushing your teeth in the morning.
  - Do another set during your morning break.
  - Do a 3rd set at lunch.
  - Do a set of exercises while reading or watching TV.
  - Do the last set when you go to bed.
- Wear a pad if you leak urine. You should stop leaking urine after you have your baby.

When do I call my doctor or nurse?

- Call if you have pain or burning when you pee.
- Call if you have pain in your lower belly.
- Call if your bladder feels very full, but you pee only a little.
- Call if you have chills or a fever.

Swollen Feet

What is it?

It is extra fluid in the feet and ankles.

What do I need to know?

- A small amount of swelling in the feet and ankles is normal. It builds up during the day. The swelling should be less in the morning.
- Swelling is worse in hot weather.
- A lot of swelling can be a sign of a problem.
- Swelling of the face or hands is not normal. Call your doctor.

What should I do?

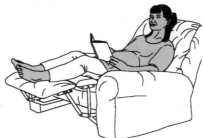

- Sit with your legs up.
- Do not stand for a long time. If you must stand, wear support panty hose.
- Do not wear socks like knee-highs with a tight elastic band. They slow the blood flow in your legs. They can cause swelling and other problems.

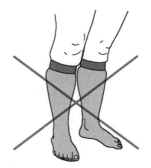

- Do not cross your legs. This stops the blood flow in your legs. It can cause more swelling and other problems.

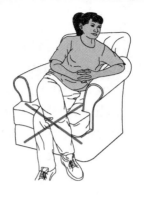

- Lie on your left side 2 times during the day, if you can. Do this while you watch TV or read. It's good for the blood flow in your legs.

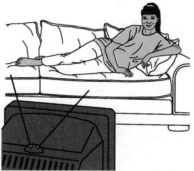

- Do not add salt to your food.
  Avoid foods that have a lot of hidden salt, like:
  - Potato chips
  - Salted nuts
  - Bacon
  - Deli meats
  - Pickles
  - Many canned soups and vegetables
  - Many vegetable juices

- Read the label to find out how much salt or sodium is in food. Avoid foods that have more than 400 mg. of sodium in a serving.

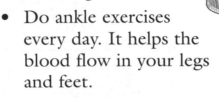

Total Fat 2g	3%	Total Carb. 8g	3%
Sat. Fat 0.5g	3%	Fiber Less than 1g	3%
Cholest. 10mg	3%	Sugars 1g	
Sodium 890mg	37%	Protein 3g	
Vitamin A 4% • Vitamin C 0% • Calcium 0% • Iron 2%			

- Do ankle exercises every day. It helps the blood flow in your legs and feet.

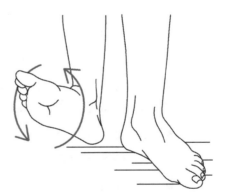

  - Sit in a chair.
  - Lift your right foot off the floor.
  - Draw a circle in the air with your toes. Do 10 circles.
  - Now do 10 circles with the same foot going the other way.
  - Put your right foot down. Lift your left foot off the floor.
  - Do 10 circles each way with your left foot.
  - Do this exercise 2 times a day.

Swollen Feet

When do I call my doctor or nurse?

- Call if you gain 2 or more pounds in one week.
- Call if you have a lot more swelling in your feet and ankles.
- Call if you have swelling in the morning.
- Call if you get swelling in your face or hands.

Other Things You May Feel

What is it?

Your growing baby changes
your body and how you feel.

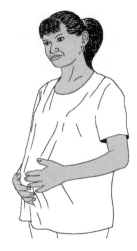

What do I need to know?

- Here are some changes you
  may have during pregnancy:
  - Feeling very tired
  - Mood swings
  - Large veins in the legs
  - Trouble sleeping
- Some women feel sick during pregnancy.
  Others feel well and have few problems.
- Being active and eating healthy food will help
  you feel your best. These things are also good for
  your baby.

What should I do?

- **Feeling very tired:**
  - You will feel tired in the first 3 months of
    pregnancy and again in the last 2 months.
  - Take it easy. Do not try to do too many things.

- Feeling very tired can be a sign that you are not eating healthy. Read what to eat on pages 25–29.

- If you work, try to work less hours. Take breaks and sit with your feet up.

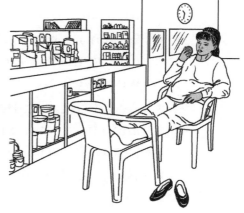

- Do less work at home.

- Listen to your body. If you feel tired, get more rest. Take a nap during the day if you can.

- Go to bed earlier. Try to get 8–10 hours of sleep each night.

- Make sure you are getting enough exercise. Walk at least 30 minutes a day.

- **Mood Swings:**

  - Mood swings means feeling happy one minute and sad the next. You may cry about silly things. You may feel anxious about being a mom. These feelings are normal. They come from the changes in your body.

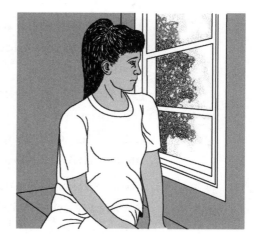

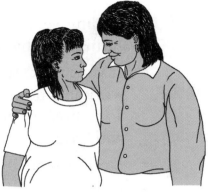

- Tell your family and friends how you feel. Ask them for their support.

- Get more rest. You can be more moody when you are tired.

- Avoid sugar, caffeine, and chocolate. They can make you feel anxious or down.

- Eat a healthy diet. Get regular exercise.

- Talk to your doctor if you have:

    - Little interest in the things you used to enjoy.

    - Changes in your eating (no appetite or you can't stop eating).

    - Trouble sleeping, or you want to sleep all the time.

- **Large veins in the legs:**

    - The veins in the legs can swell. This is called varicose veins.

    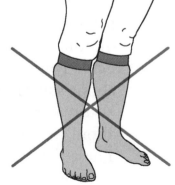

    - Do not wear socks that are tight around your legs. This can stop the blood flow in your legs.

    - Wear support panty hose if you stand or walk a lot. Put the hose on before you get out of bed in the morning.

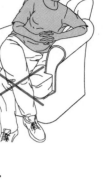

- Do not sit with your legs crossed. This is bad for the blood flow in your legs.

- Avoid standing or sitting in one place for a long time. Put your feet up when sitting.

- Get regular exercise, like walking. It's good for the blood flow in your legs.

- Read about swollen feet on pages 104–107.

- **Trouble sleeping:**

  - Get some exercise during the day. Do not exercise within 3 hours of going to bed.

  - Do relaxing things before going to bed, like:
    - ◆ Reading
    - ◆ Taking a warm (not hot) bath
    - ◆ Hugging and kissing

  - Avoid things that have caffeine. These include coffee, tea, chocolate, and some sodas.

  - Do not take sleeping pills.

  - Eat a light snack and drink a glass of warm milk before going to bed.

  - Try to clear your mind of worries.

  - It's hard to get comfortable during the last 3 months of pregnancy. Lie on your side with a pillow under your stomach and between your legs.

- Drink your 8–10 glasses of fluid before 5 p.m. Do this so you do not have to get up many times at night to pee.

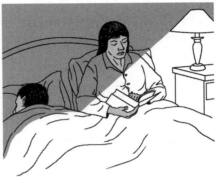

- If you can't sleep, read a book or watch TV. Do this until you feel sleepy. Do not worry about not being able to sleep. It will not hurt you or your baby.

When do I call my doctor or nurse?

- Call before you take any medicines your doctor did not order. This includes over-the-counter medicines, like vitamins and herbs.
- Call if you want to know if what you are feeling is normal.

More Things to Know 5

Notes

_____

_____

_____

_____

_____

_____

_____

_____

_____

_____

_____

_____

_____

_____

_____

Safety Tips

What is it?

Things to do to avoid getting hurt.

What do I need to know?

- The same safety rules apply to pregnant women as to everyone else. Always be careful when walking, driving, working, and cleaning.

- Your body shape changes during pregnancy. This can make you unstable. It's easy for you to slip and fall.

- Pregnant women can feel dizzy or faint. If you feel dizzy or faint, sit down right away. If you are driving, pull over to the side of the road.

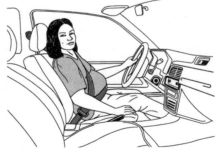

- Pregnant women should wear car seat belts. The lap belt should be worn under the belly.

- Pregnant women should avoid using harsh cleansers. They give off fumes that can be harmful.

- Pregnant women should not wash the inside of their vagina with water. This is called a douche.

- Do not take hot baths or exercise too hard. It's bad to get your body very hot when you are pregnant.

- Do not take hot baths or sit in hot tubs or steam baths. Your bath water should feel only a little warmer than your skin.

- Some pregnant women are hit or hurt by their partners. This is abuse. This can cause early labor or loss of the baby. You must tell your doctor or nurse.

- Women need to get help to stop the abuse. There is a 24 hour hotline women can call for help. The number is 1-800-799-7233 or 1-800-787-3224 TTY.

- The front of the phone book also lists places women can call for help. They need to look under Child Abuse and Family Violence.

What should I do?

- Get help if your partner hits or hurts you.
  Talk to your doctor or call 1-800-799-7233.

- Always wear a seat belt when riding in a car.
  Place the lap belt as low as you can under your belly.
  Place the shoulder belt over the shoulder and across the center of your chest. Do not put it behind your head or under your arm.

- Never climb on a chair or ladder.

- Do not lift heavy things.
  If you must lift, bend and lift from the knees.
  Keep your back straight.

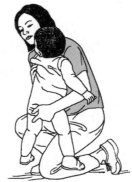

- Hold on to something when bending or getting up.

- Wear flat shoes that fit well. Do not wear high heels.

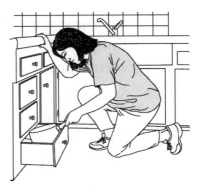

- Keep the floor clear of phone cords and other things you can trip over. Remove rugs that you can slide on.

- Hold on to handrails when climbing up or down stairs.

- Do not douche. This is not safe to do when pregnant.

- Use rubber mats in the bathtub and shower. Be careful when getting in and out of the tub or shower.

- Avoid walking on ice or snow.

MAT→

- Get 8–10 hours of sleep a night. Do not push yourself to do things when you feel tired. Rest when you feel tired.

- Wash your hands often. Wash your hands after touching raw meat and pets.

- Do not clean the cat litter. You can get an illness that can harm your baby.

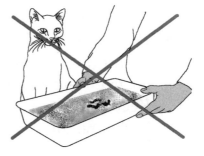

- Do not touch pet hamsters or guinea pigs. They can carry disease that can harm your baby. Get others to care for the pet and clean the cage.

- Get help if you have rats or mice around the house.

When do I call my doctor or nurse?

- Call if you have questions about something you want to do.

- Call if you had a fall or an accident.

- Call if your partner hits or hurts you.

- There is a 24 hour hotline women can call for help. The number is 1-800-799-7233 or 1-800-787-3224 TTY.

- The front of the phone book also lists places under Child Abuse and Family Violence that women can call for help.

Early Labor

What is it?

Early labor is labor that starts 3 or more weeks before you are due.

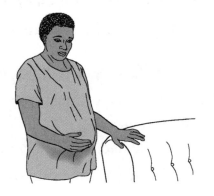

What do I need to know?

- Babies need 40 weeks to grow. A baby is not ready to be born before 37 weeks.

- Early labor is bad. Babies born early are often very small and sick.

- There is medicine that can stop early labor. It needs to be given right away. It can stop a baby from being born too early.

- Here are some warning signs of early labor:

  - The uterus starts to tighten (feels hard). This happens every 10–15 minutes or more often. This is called having contractions. Contractions make the cervix open so the baby can pass.

  - Cramps in your belly as if you are starting your period

  - Dull lower back pain. It is not the same as your normal backache.

- Pressure in your pelvis that feels like the baby is pushing down
- Thick vaginal discharge with some blood
- Fluid leaking or gushing from your vagina
- A feeling that something is not right

- Some things can cause early labor, like:
  - Smoking or being around someone who smokes
  - Drinking alcohol like wine, beer, or hard liquor
  - Taking street drugs like cocaine, marijuana, and uppers
  - Being hit or abused
  - Taking medicines without your doctor's OK
  - Falls and other accidents
  - Very hard work or exercise
  - Taking hot baths
  - Taking laxatives
  - Rubbing your nipples
  - High fever
  - High blood pressure

What should I do?

- Avoid things that can make you go into labor early.
- If you think you may be having contractions, do these things:
  - Stop what you are doing.
  - Go pee.

- Drink 2 glasses of water.
- Lie down. Put your hands on your belly. Feel for contractions.
- Count each time your uterus gets hard and then soft. This is one contraction. Count how many contractions you have in an hour.

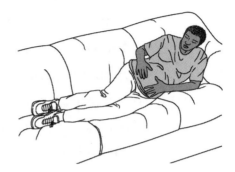

- Call your doctor if:
    - You have more than 4 contractions in 1 hour, or
    - You have any of the warning signs listed on pages 118–119.

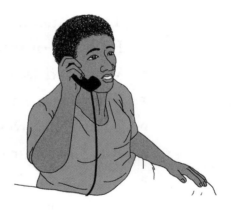

- Call your doctor right away. Do not wait to see what happens.
- Your doctor will ask you questions like:
    - Do you have any cramping or pain?
    - How often do you feel contractions?
    - Do you have any fluid coming out of your vagina?
    - Do you have any bleeding?

- Your doctor may tell you to lie down on your left side for 1 hour and drink 4 glasses of water.

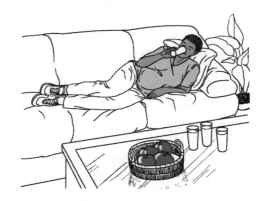

- Your doctor may tell you to come to the office or go to the hospital.

- Do what your doctor tells you.

When do I call my doctor or nurse?

- Call if you have signs of early labor.
- Call if you are not sure if what you are feeling is normal.

Working Moms

What is it?

Many pregnant
women work
outside the home.
There are things
you can do to keep
your baby safe.

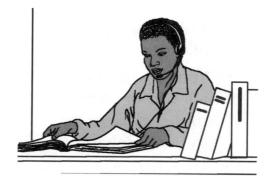

What do I need to know?

- Most healthy women are able to work while they are pregnant. Many women work up to the time they have the baby.

- There are many kinds of jobs. Some jobs have risks. Risks are things that can hurt you or your baby. Some risks are:

  - Working with metals like lead and other poisons

  - Working with chemicals or fumes

  - Working near x-rays

  - Heavy lifting and other hard work

  - Working with machines that shake or are heavy

  - Working more than 8 hours a day

  - A changing work shift (working days, then nights, then back to days)

- A lot of stress
- Working where there is very loud noise or in a very hot or cold place

- Your doctor can tell you if your work has risks to you or your baby.

- People at work can help you if your job has risks. They may need to change the job you do to protect your baby.

- You can't be fired from your job just because you are pregnant. There are laws that make sure you do not get fired. Check with your local Employment Office to find out about these laws. You can also call 1-800-669-4000 to find out about your rights. This is the number to the Equal Employment Opportunity Commission.

- If you get sick and can't work, you may be able to get disability benefits or unemployment. You may get money during the time you are not working. Find out about your benefits at work. You can also call or go to your local employment office.

- The Family Medical Leave Act is a law that allows you to take time off work if you are sick and after you have your baby. You can take time off and still keep your job. Laws change, so check with your boss.

- If you need help, speak with a social worker. You can find one at your health care clinic or at the hospital where you will have your baby.

What should I do?

- Tell your doctor about your job and what you do. Talk about any risks and what to do about them.

- Read your work's rules about pregnancy. Learn about your state's laws about pregnancy and work. Know your rights before you tell your boss that you are pregnant.

- Talk with your doctor and your family about how much time you will need to take off work.

- Let your boss know how much time off you will need. Let your boss know when you will return to work.

- Try to rest a few times during the day. If you stand most of the time, sit down during lunch and on breaks. Read what to do for back pain on pages 90–94.

- Use your car to rest if there is no other place. If you do not have a car, ask someone if you can use their car.

- Try to put your feet up as much as you can. Put a pillow under your feet.

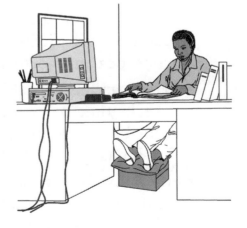

- Wear support stockings made for pregnant women. They help the blood flow in your legs. Put them on before you get out of bed in the morning. Ask your doctor to order them. Your health insurance may pay for them.

- Wear flat shoes that feel good.

- Stretch your legs once every 30 minutes. Do ankle exercises every 2–3 hours.

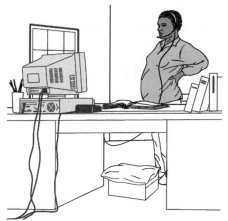

- If you sit most of the day, try to stand and walk around for 2–3 minutes each hour.

- Bring a sweater to work. Take it off if you get hot. Put it on if you feel cold.

- If you work with metals or chemicals, be sure to talk to your doctor about the risks to your baby.

- Do not lift heavy things. Ask for help if you need it.

- Do not climb ladders. Do not do things that can cause you to fall.

- If you are asked to do something you think can hurt you or your baby, do not do it. Talk to your boss about it. Be sure to tell your doctor about it.

When do I call my doctor or nurse?

- Call if you want to know if your work is safe.

- Call if you are asked to do something at work that you think can hurt you or your baby.

- Call if you need to speak to a social worker about your rights.

Sex During Pregnancy

What is it?

It is having sex or making love during the time you are pregnant.

What do I need to know?

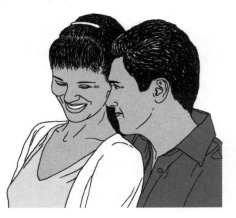

- Love and affection are important during pregnancy.
- Pregnancy changes how a woman feels about sex. A woman's sex drive may go up or down. It's not the same for all women or all pregnancies.
- Some people find sex better during this time because they do not have to worry about getting pregnant.
- Some people worry about hurting the baby during sex.
- Sex during pregnancy is safe if the woman is not having any problems. You **must not** have sex after your water breaks. You need to go to the hospital after your water breaks.
- Pregnant women should not lay flat on their back after the 4th month. It is bad for the blood flow.

Sex During Pregnancy

What should I do?

- Talk with your doctor if you have any questions about sex.
- Talk to your doctor before having sex if:

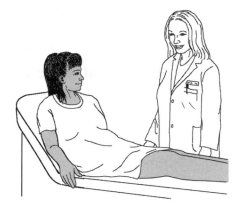

  - You lost a baby in a past pregnancy.
  - You had a baby early in a past pregnancy.
  - You or your partner has a sexually transmitted disease (STD).
  - You are having vaginal bleeding.
  - You have pain during sex.
  - You are having problems with your pregnancy.
  - You have been told that the placenta (afterbirth) is in the wrong place.

- You can have sex as often as you want unless your doctor tells you not to. Use positions that do not press on your belly. Do not lay flat on your back after the 4th month.

- Show love in other ways if you can't or do not feel like having sex. Give lots of hugs and kisses. Give back and foot rubs. Touch each other in tender ways.

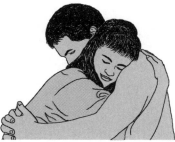

- Talk with your partner about how you feel. Be open and honest.
- Stop having sex and call your doctor if you have bleeding, or pain, or if your water breaks.

When do I call my doctor or nurse?

- Call if you have questions about sex.

Getting a Cold or the Flu

What is it?

Many women get a
cold or the flu while
they are pregnant.

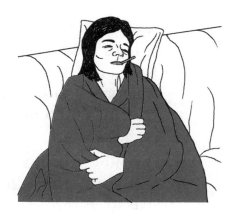

What do I need to know?

- Pregnant women should
  ask their doctor before
  getting a flu shot.

- People catch more colds when they are tired or
  run down.

- Colds and flu are caused by a virus. There is no
  medicine to kill a virus.

- Antibiotics do not work on colds or the flu because
  they do not kill viruses.

- The best thing a pregnant woman can do is stay away
  from people who are sick.

- A cold or the flu can last from 8–10 days.

- Some signs of a cold or the flu are:
  - Sneezing
  - Watery eyes
  - Headache
  - Muscle aches

- Fever
- Loss of appetite
- You can get a high fever with a cold or flu. A high fever can hurt your baby. Call your doctor if you have a fever of 100.6 degrees F or higher.

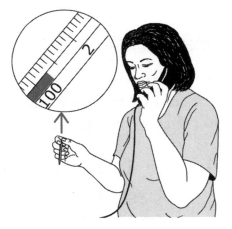

- A cold or the flu can turn into other illnesses like strep throat.

What should I do?

- Try to stay well. Get lots of rest. Eat healthy foods, and drink 8–10 glasses of fluids a day.
- Ask your doctor if you should get a flu shot.
- Wash your hands often. Keep your hands away from your face.
- Wash your hands before eating.
- Do not share food or drinks with other people.

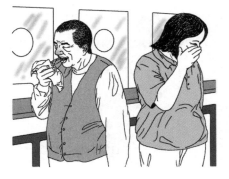

- Stay away from people who sneeze or cough. Turn your head away if someone sneezes or coughs.

- If you feel like you are getting sick, rest more. Drink more fluids.
- If you get a cold, rest in bed. Eat as much as you can. Drink 10–12 glasses of fluids.
- If you have a stuffy nose, use a cool mist machine (humidifier).
- If you have a fever:
  - Take a cool shower or bath.
  - Wear clothes that keep you cool.
  - Drink lots of cool fluids.
- Do not take any medicine unless your doctor says it's OK.
- Ask your doctor if you can take Tylenol to bring down your fever.

When do I call my doctor or nurse?

- Call if you have a red rash.
- Call if you have a fever of 100.6 degrees F or higher.
- Call if you have pain in your ears, or a sore throat.
- Call if you have white or yellow spots on the back of your throat.
- Call if you are coughing up thick green or yellow stuff.
- Call if you have other signs like many watery bowel movements (diarrhea), throwing up, or pain when you pee.
- Call if you are not well after 8 days.
- Call if you have to stay in bed and cannot go to work.

Losing the Baby

What is it?

It is the loss of a pregnancy. The baby dies inside or comes out too early and cannot live.

What do I need to know?

- Sometimes the baby dies inside. This can happen early or late in the pregnancy.
- Sometimes the baby comes out too early. This is called having a miscarriage. It can happen anytime during the first 20 weeks of pregnancy.
- Signs of a possible miscarriage are:
  - Vaginal bleeding with cramps in the lower belly
  - Blood clots or pink or gray tissue coming out of the vagina
  - Bad stomach pain
  - A lot of bleeding
  - Spotting for 3 days
- A woman needs to call her doctor if she has signs of losing the baby.
- Many times the reason for losing the baby is not known. Some women lose more than one baby.
- These things can cause a woman to lose a baby:
  - Smoking, drinking alcohol, or taking drugs

- A high fever or infection
- Taking medicines harmful to the baby
- A bad fall or other accident

- Some women are hit or hurt by their partner. This is called abuse. It can cause a woman to lose her baby.

- Women often feel ashamed and try to hide the abuse. They need to get help to protect themselves and their unborn baby. There is a 24 hour hotline women can call for help. The number is 1-800-799-7233 or 1-800-787-3224 TTY.

- The front of the phone book also lists places to call for help (see Child Abuse and Family Violence).

- A woman needs to wait 3 months after losing a baby before trying to get pregnant again.

What should I do?

- If you are having a little vaginal bleeding, lie down and rest. You may not be losing the baby. Stop having sex until bleeding has stopped for 3 days.

- If you have signs of a miscarriage or think you had a miscarriage, see your doctor.

- If anything comes out of your vagina, put it in a jar. Take it to your doctor.

- Get help if your partner hits or hurts you. Talk to your doctor about what you can do.

When do I call my doctor or nurse?

- Call if your baby moves less than before or not at all.
- Call if you think you are losing the baby.
- Call if you were hurt or were in an accident.
- Call for help if your partner hits or hurts you.
  Check the front of the phone book under Child Abuse and Family Violence or call 1-800-799-7233 or 1-800-787-3224 TTY.

The Birth of Your Baby 6

Notes

Labor

What is it?

Labor is having contractions of the uterus that get harder and come often. They push the baby down and open the cervix.

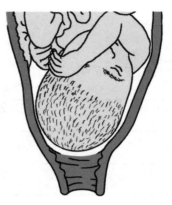

What do I need to know?

- Labor is a natural thing leading to the birth of a baby.

- It's helpful to have someone with you during labor and delivery. This person can be the baby's father, a family member, or a friend. This person is your labor partner or coach. He or she will:
    - Comfort you
    - Time your contractions
    - Help you to breathe during contractions
    - Remind you to rest between contractions

- A woman's body starts to get ready for labor in the last month of pregnancy.

- Some women go into labor slowly. They have mild cramps or back pain.

Labor

- Labor can start fast with a gush of clear fluid from the vagina. This happens when the bag of water around the baby (amniotic sac) breaks.

- Once the water breaks, a woman can get an infection. She needs to go to the hospital right away. She should not take a bath or put anything into the vagina.

- At first, contractions come every 15–20 minutes. They last 30–45 seconds. Contractions get stronger and closer as labor goes on if it is **real** labor.

- Sometimes the contractions come and go. This is called "false labor." Wait for them to get regular and closer together again.

- Many women spend the early part of labor at home. They walk around and watch TV to pass the time. Walking around is good. It helps the baby move down. Taking a shower or bath helps you feel better.

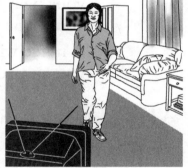

- Your doctor will tell you when to go to the hospital. You may be told to go when your contractions are 5–10 minutes apart and 1 minute long.

- Here is a list of warning signs that something may be wrong. Go to the hospital right away if you have any of these signs:
    - Green colored fluid coming from the vagina
    - Bleeding from the vagina like a period
    - Baby moves less or not at all.

- Here's what happens when you get to the hospital:
  - You will go to a special place in the hospital called labor and delivery.
  - The nurse will check your temperature, blood pressure, and pulse.
  - A doctor or nurse will do a pelvic exam to check your cervix. This tells how close you are to delivery.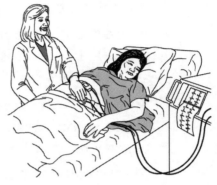
  - A device will be put on your belly to check your baby's heart rate.
  - A nurse will watch how you and your baby are doing.

What should I do?

- Call your labor partner when labor starts.
- Make sure you have a ride to the hospital.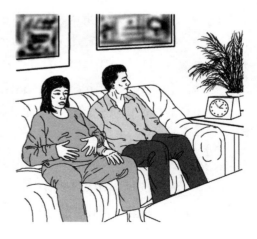
- Count how often your contractions come and how long they last:
  - Put your hands on your belly.
  - Feel your belly get hard.

- Count how many seconds it takes for your belly to get soft. That's how long the contraction lasted.
- The number of minutes that pass before your belly starts to get hard again is how far apart your contractions are.

- Walk around, squat, or sit. These positions help your baby to move down.
- Play a game or watch a movie to pass the time.
- Ask your doctor if it's OK to eat and drink.
- Use breathing to help when contractions get stronger. Breathe slowly in through your mouth and nose. Purse your lips and blow the air out slowly.
- Go to the hospital when your doctor tells you.
- Go to the hospital right away if:
  - You have heavy bleeding from your vagina like a period.
  - Your water breaks.
  - You have green colored fluid leaking from your vagina.
  - Baby moves less or not at all.

When do I call my doctor or nurse?

- Call if you are in labor and you do not know what to do.
- Call if you have a question or feel that something is wrong.
- Go to the hospital if you have one or more warning signs listed above.

Delivery

What is it?

It is the birth of your baby.

What do I need to know?

- When your cervix is open all the way, you will feel like pushing.

- When the top of your baby's head shows, your doctor may make a small cut at the opening of your vagina. This is called an episiotomy. The cut makes the opening bigger for your baby to pass through.

- You will push only when the doctor or nurse tells you to. You will do this until your baby is born. This is called having a vaginal delivery.

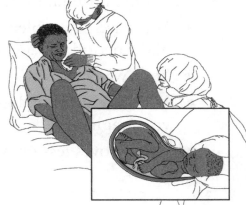

- Most women have vaginal deliveries.

- Some women need to have their baby delivered through the belly. This is called a C-section.

- Here are some reasons why a C-section is done:
  - Baby is in the wrong position.
  - Baby's head is too big to pass.
  - Baby is sick.
  - Labor is too hard on baby and the cervix does not open.
  - Mom has a certain sexually transmitted disease (STD).
- You will feel tired but happy after your baby is born.

What should I do?

- Listen to your doctor and labor partner.
  Do what they say.
- Rest between contractions.
- Focus on your breathing.
- Push only when your doctor tells you to push.

After Your Baby Is Born

7

Notes

How You Feel

What is it?

It's the first few days after your baby is born.
You may feel happy and sad at the same time.
You may feel sore all over.

What do I need to know?

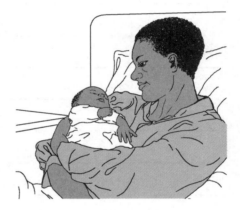

- You may feel very tired right after you give birth. You worked hard. Many new moms just want to sleep.

- Some moms want to hold and feed their baby right away.

- Some new moms feel a little down or blue. This can happen from the changes in the body after giving birth. Moms feel better by talking about their feelings with a friend. Going out every day for a walk helps. The sad feelings get less and go away within 10 days of giving birth. This is called baby blues.

- Some women feel very depressed. They are not able to take care of themselves or their baby. This is called postpartum depression. Women with postpartum depression need help from a doctor. Some need to take medicine to feel better.

- Some moms are scared about taking care of their baby. They are not sure what to do. These feelings are normal. Do not be afraid to ask for help.

- Most new moms have a sore bottom from the stitches and cramps in their belly. This is called after pains.

- Here are other body changes and discomforts new moms have:
  - Vaginal bleeding lasting 2–6 weeks. It's heavy the first few days and then it's light.
  - Constipation
  - Hemorrhoids
  - Sore breasts
  - Tired and sore all over
  - Sweating a lot

- Some women get infections and other problems after delivery. Here are warning signs of a problem. Call your doctor right away if you have:
  - Heavy vaginal bleeding. You soak one or more pads in 1 hour.
  - Vaginal fluid that smells bad
  - Fever of 100 degrees F or higher
  - Throwing up or you can't eat
  - Pain or burning when you pee
  - Redness or pain in your legs
  - Red streaks or tender spots on your breasts
  - Severe headaches

- New moms need to get up and move around.
  - It's good for the blood flow in the legs.
  - It helps constipation.
  - It helps the body get back to normal.

What should I do?

- Sit in warm water 2 or 3 times a day. This will help the soreness around your vagina and hemorrhoids. Your doctor may order some cream for the hemorrhoids. Read what to do for hemorrhoids on pages 99–100.

- Drink 8–10 glasses of fluid a day. It helps you to have a bowel movement. Read about other things to do for constipation on pages 95–98.

- You need a lot of rest. Take naps during the day. Take a nap when your baby naps.

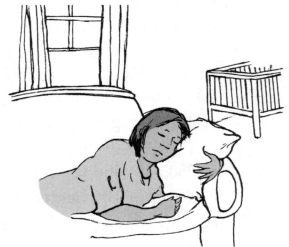

- Your doctor can order medicine for pain. It's OK to take Tylenol.

- Be sure to walk around.

- Wear a bra that fits well. This will help your sore breasts.

- Use ice packs for sore breasts if you are not breastfeeding. Put warm packs on your breasts if you are breastfeeding.

- Avoid having sex until you see your doctor. If you have sex, be sure to use a condom or other form of birth control. You can get pregnant after having a baby. This can happen even if you are breastfeeding.

- See your doctor 4–6 weeks after you give birth. Your doctor will check that you are healed. Talk with your doctor about birth control if you do not know what to use.

When do I call my doctor or nurse?

- Call if you have one or more warning signs listed on page 145.

- Call if you do not feel like eating or are not able to sleep.

- Call if you cry all the time and are not able to take care of yourself or your baby.

- Call if you feel mad at your baby or you do not feel like taking care of your baby.

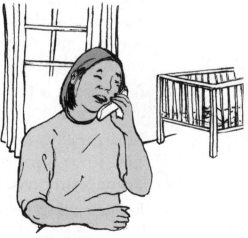

- Call if you feel like you want to hit your baby. If you feel this way, put your baby down and walk away. Call someone for help.

- Call to see your doctor 4–6 weeks after you have your baby.

Feeding Your Baby

What is it?

Your new baby can be breastfed or bottle-fed.

What do I need to know?

- There are many good reasons to breastfeed like:
  - Breast milk is healthy for your baby. It has all the right things for your baby.

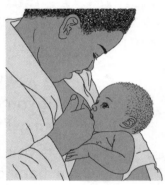

  - It helps your baby fight infection in the first few months of life. Breastfed babies tend to get sick less than bottle-fed babies and have less risk of other childhood problems like diabetes, obesity, and cancer.
  - Breast milk is free. You can save over $1,000 by breastfeeding your baby for 6 months.
  - Breast milk is easy to give to your baby. It does not have to be warmed or put into a bottle. There is no cleanup after feeding.
  - Breastfeeding helps you lose weight. Women who breastfeed get their shape back faster than women who bottle-feed.
- It is best to breastfeed your baby for 1 year, but any time is better than none.

- If you breastfeed, you will need nursing bras and pads.

- You do not need to have large breasts to breastfeed. Even if your breasts are small, your body will make as much milk as your baby needs.

- Breastfeeding does not stop a woman from getting pregnant. It is not a form of birth control.

- Women who breastfeed need to take their vitamins. They also need to eat the same amount of food like when they were pregnant.

- There are programs to help nursing mothers get the healthy food they need. It's called the WIC (women, infants, and children) program. You can get information about WIC from your doctor's office or by calling WIC. You can find the number for WIC in the front of the phone book under Mother and Infant Health.

- Women who work can still breastfeed. They may need to rent a breast pump. An electric pump works best. Some insurance pays for renting breast pumps.

- Women can pump their breasts anytime. They need to put the milk in the refrigerator or freezer for later use. Breast milk is good for 72 hours in the refrigerator or 3 months in the freezer.

- **Things to know about bottle feeding:**
  - Some women cannot breastfeed. They may be sick or taking medicine for an illness.
  - Some women can't or do not want to breastfeed. This is OK. The baby will be fine.

- If you are bottle feeding, wear a tight bra. Do not try to get milk out of your breasts.

- You can put ice packs on your breasts and take Tylenol for pain.

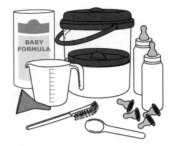

- You will need bottles, brushes, nipples, and baby formula.

- Your doctor will tell you which formula is right for your baby.

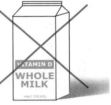

- **Use baby formula, not cow's milk.**

- Make the formula the right way. Some formula is ready to feed. Some formula needs to be mixed with water. Read on the can how to mix the formula.

- If you need to add water to make the formula, be sure to add the right amount.

  - If you use too much water, the formula will be too weak. Your baby will be hungry and cry a lot.

  - If you do not add enough water, the formula will be too strong. It will make your baby very sick.

- Keep the formula you mix in the refrigerator. Your baby will get sick if the formula is not kept cold.

- If you do not use the mixed formula within 48 hours, throw it away.

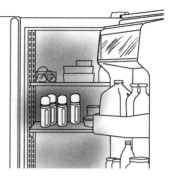

- Throw away any formula left in the bottle after each feeding.

- Wash bottles and nipples with soap and hot water. Rinse well.

- Bottle-feeding allows the father to feed the baby.

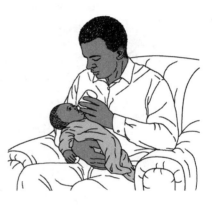

What should I do?

Breastfeeding:

- Breastfeeding gets easier after the first few days. You may have some trouble at first. This is normal. You and your baby need to learn. Early milk is called colostrum. It is very good for your baby.

- The nurses at the hospital can teach you how to breastfeed. Ask for help while you are in the hospital. Get a phone number to call for help after you get home.

- Wash your hands before you breastfeed.

- You can learn to breastfeed your baby.

Step 1:

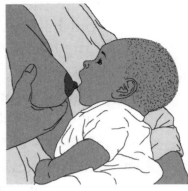

- Turn baby's head toward your breast.

- Hold the breast with your thumb on top and fingers below.

- Touch baby's lower lip with your nipple. This makes baby open his mouth.

Step 2:

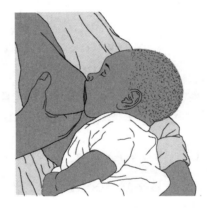

- Put your nipple in when baby opens his mouth.

- Baby's lips should cover most of the dark part of the nipple. Baby's tongue should be under the nipple.

- Hold baby close to you.

- Feed for at least 10–15 minutes on each breast.

Step 3:

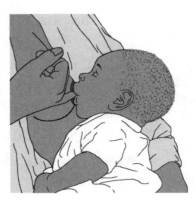

- To change breasts, put your little finger in the corner of baby's mouth. This breaks the seal.

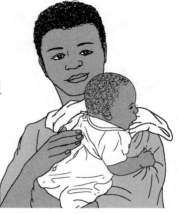

- Burp your baby. Hold your baby over your shoulder. Gently rub or pat baby's back.

- A breastfed baby does not need to be burped as often as a bottle-fed baby.

- Repeat steps 1 and 2 with your other breast. Baby will take less milk from this breast, so start the next feeding with this breast.

• Your baby needs to breastfeed at least 8 times a day. This means you need to feed your baby every 2–3 hours. You may need to wake your baby up for a feeding.

• Your baby should have 6 to 8 wet diapers a day. If your baby has that many wet diapers, he or she is getting enough milk.

6 to 8 Diapers

• Things you eat or drink may pass to your baby through your breast milk. Some foods can make your baby cranky. If your baby gets cranky, stop eating these foods for 2 weeks:

- Chocolate, coffee, and other things with caffeine

- Spicy foods

- Foods that cause gas, like beans

- Do not take any medicine while you are breastfeeding unless your doctor says it's OK.

- Wash your breasts with warm water every day. Do not use soap on your breasts. Soap can cause your nipples to get dry and crack. Let your nipples air-dry.

- Ask your doctor or nurse about special cream to put on your nipples if they are cracked or sore.

- If you need to pump your breasts, call the 800 number of your health insurance. Your insurance may pay for the cost of the rental. They will tell you where to get the pump.

- If your insurance does not pay for renting a breast pump, call the nurse at the hospital to find out where to rent a pump. The place where you rent the pump will have someone teach you how to use it. Get a phone number to call if you have more questions about breast pumping.

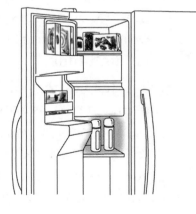

- If you use a breast pump, be sure to put the pumped milk in the refrigerator or freezer.

Bottle feeding:

- Your doctor will tell you which formula to buy. You can buy formula at a food market or drugstore.

- Wash your hands before you mix the formula.

- Mix the baby formula just as it says on the can. Some formulas need to be mixed with water. Some formulas are ready to use. You do not need to add water. Ask someone to help you if you do not know what to do.

- Hold your baby upright during feedings. Do not feed your baby lying flat:

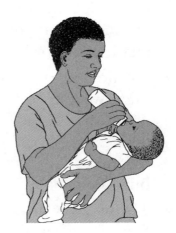

  - Your baby can choke if you feed him lying down.

  - Formula can run into your baby's ears and cause an infection.

- Never prop the bottle or leave your baby alone with the bottle. Your baby can choke.

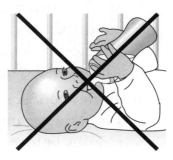

- Do not put your baby to bed with a bottle.

- A new baby needs to get 16–24 ounces of formula a day. The amount depends on how big your baby is. Feed your baby 2–3 ounces at each feeding. Your baby needs to feed every 3–4 hours. Call the nurse at the hospital if you have questions.

- Warm the bottle in a bowl of hot water. Test how warm the formula is. Do this by putting a few drops on your inside wrist. It should feel warm, not hot.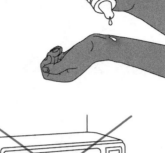

- **Do not** use a microwave to warm the bottle. The hot formula can burn your baby.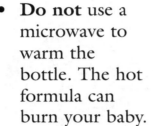

- Throw away any formula left in the bottle after feeding your baby.

- Wash the bottles and nipples with hot, soapy water. Use a brush to clean the insides of the bottles. Rinse the bottles and nipples well. Your baby can get sick if he or she drinks from a bottle that has soap in it.

- Wash new bottles and boil new nipples 5 minutes before you use them.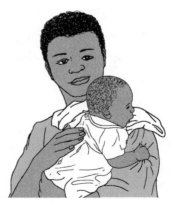

- Burp your baby after every 1–2 ounces of feeding. Hold your baby up over your shoulder. Gently rub or pat baby's back.

- If your baby is fussy or cries a lot, try burping your baby after every ½–1 ounce.
- Bring your baby to see the doctor when the doctor tells you. This is around 1 or 2 weeks after you bring the baby home.
- Whether you breast or bottle-feed your baby, you need to eat a healthy diet. Drink 8–10 glasses of fluids a day.
- Rest as much as you can.
- See your doctor 4–6 weeks after you have your baby.

When do I call my doctor or nurse?

- Call if your baby refuses 2 feedings in a row.
- Call if your baby does not have at least 6 wet diapers in 24 hours.
- Call if your baby's temperature taken under the arm is 100 degrees F or higher.
- Call if your baby does not have 1 bowel movement within 24 hours after birth.
- Call if you feel burning or pain in your breasts.
- Call if your breasts have red streaks or hard lumps.
- Call if you have sore, red nipples or cracks or blisters on your nipples.
- Call if you have questions or need help with feeding.
- Call if you feel mad at your baby or you do not feel like taking care of your baby.
- Call if you feel like you want to hurt yourself or your baby.

The First Few Days
with Your Baby

What is it?

A new baby changes the way things are done. He or she affects everyone in the family.

What do I need to know?

- The nurses at the hospital teach new moms how to care for their babies. New moms need to learn how to:
    - Hold a baby
    - Feed a baby
    - Burp a baby
    - Change diapers
    - Bathe a baby
    - Care for baby's belly button
    - Care for a baby boy's penis after circumcision
- It's a law that a baby has to be put in an infant car seat when riding in a car. Make sure you have a car seat. Tell the nurse at the hospital, if you do not have a car seat. Some hospitals give away free car seats.

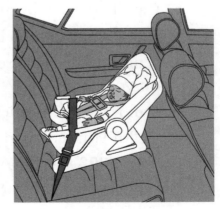

The First Few Days with Your Baby

- New babies can sleep 16–18 hours a day. They may wake often and then go back to sleep.

- A baby may have the hiccups or sneeze. This is normal.

- Babies cry to tell you they need something. Babies cry to tell you they:

  - Are hungry.
  - Need a diaper change.
  - Want to be held and rocked.
  - Have gas pains.
  - Are too hot or too cold.
  - Are tired.

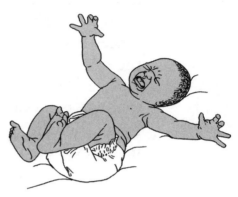

- Some babies cry more than others. It does not mean you are a bad parent if your baby cries a lot. Try feeding your baby more often. Burp your baby after every ½–1 ounce of formula or after each breast.

- A baby needs to be held and played with when awake. Here are some things you can do:

  - Play soft music for your baby to hear
  - Talk and sing to your baby
  - Show your baby things around the house

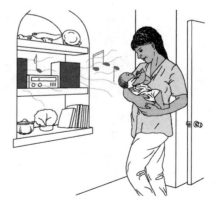

- Read stories to your baby

- Hold and rock your baby

- Here are some safety tips for your new baby:

  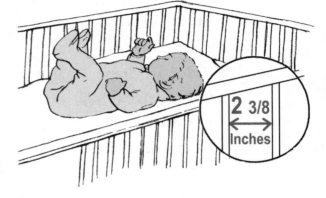

  - Use a crib that's in good condition. The spaces between the crib bars must be less than 2⅜ inches. Make sure the mattress is firm.

  - Never put a baby down on a waterbed, or pillow.

  - Do not put your baby to sleep in your bed or another child's bed.

  - Do not put pillows, stuffed animals, or toys in the crib.

  - Do not use bumper pads in the crib.

  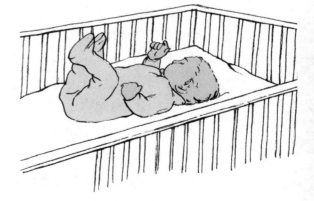

  - Do not put your baby to sleep on his or her stomach or side. Babies should sleep on their back.

- Always put your baby in a car seat when riding in a car. Do this even if you are going only 1 or 2 blocks.

  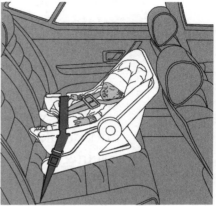

  - Use an approved infant car seat. Do not use a baby seat you use in the house.

  - Put baby in the back seat of the car. Never put baby in the front seat of the car.

  - Install the car seat facing the back of the car and leaning halfway back.

  - Be sure to install the car seat the right way. Follow the instructions that come with the car seat. Get help if you are not sure how to install the seat.

- Never leave your baby alone in a car, even for a few minutes. Always take your baby with you when you leave the car.

- Never put your baby to bed with a bottle.

  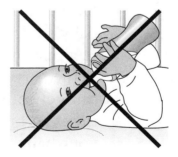

  - Your baby could choke and die.

  - Drinking milk while lying down can cause ear infections.

  - It will rot your baby's teeth when he's older.

The First Few Days with Your Baby

- Never leave your baby alone anywhere. An adult always has to be with your baby.

- Do not tie a pacifier or anything else around your baby's neck. He or she could choke.

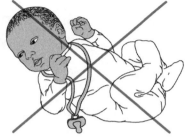

- Check your baby's pacifier every day for cuts and breaks. Buy a new pacifier every 2–3 months. Never use a bottle nipple as a pacifier.

- Do not leave your baby alone on a sofa, changing table, or other high place. Your baby can have a bad fall.

- Do not hold your baby while cooking or drinking a hot liquid like coffee.

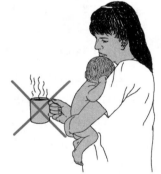

- Do not heat baby's bottle in a microwave. Some parts can get so hot they can burn your baby.

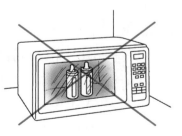

- Never hit or shake your baby. Your baby can die. If you feel angry because your baby won't stop crying, put your baby down and walk away. Call someone for help.

What should I do?

- Bathe, change baby's diaper, hold, feed, and do all the care for your baby before you leave the hospital. Get a phone number of a nurse at the hospital to call if you have questions.

- Many hospitals have a program that sends a nurse to visit new moms and babies a few days after they get home. Ask to have a visit. Be ready with questions when the nurse comes.

- Try to get help with house work so you can care for your baby and rest. Ask your mother, sister, aunt, or friend to help.

- See if the baby's father can get a few days off work to help.

- Try to keep your baby up during the day. Your baby may sleep longer during the night.

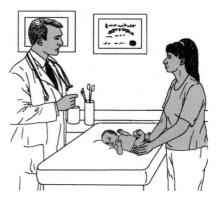

- Bring your baby to see the doctor when the doctor tells you.

- Be sure to wake your baby every 3–4 hours for feedings.
- Read and follow the safety tips on pages 160–163.
- Here's how to care for your baby's belly button:

  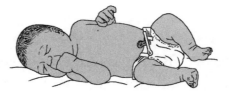

  - Do not get the belly button wet. Keep it dry until the cord falls off. Keep the diaper below the belly button.

  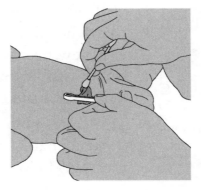

  - Clean around the belly button with 70% rubbing alcohol on a Q-tip or cotton ball. Do this every time you change the diaper.

  - Lift the cord and clean right where it meets the body. You will not hurt your baby. The alcohol does not sting. Your baby may cry because the alcohol feels cold. The cord falls off after about a week.

  - Do not put powder or oil on or around the belly button.

- If your son had the loose skin covering the tip of his penis removed (circumcision), you will learn at the hospital how to take care of it. Call if you have questions or if your baby has these signs:

  - A bad smell from around the penis
  - Yellow/green oozing

- Red and swollen penis
- Penis is not healed after 8 days.

• Hold your baby a lot. Your baby can see you best 12–14 inches away. Talk and sing to your baby. Get your baby to know your voice and your touch.

• If the weather is nice, take your baby for a walk in a stroller. Cover your baby if it is cool. Keep the sun off your baby at all times.

• Pacifiers are nipples that allow a baby to suck without feeding. Babies like to suck. Give your baby a pacifier if he or she needs one. Never use a bottle nipple as a pacifier.

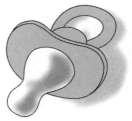

• If you are breastfeeding, try not to use a pacifier for 3 weeks so your baby can get used to your breast.

• Babies should have 6–8 wet diapers in 24 hours.

• Do not forget to take care of yourself. Get lots of rest. Eat healthy foods and drink lots of fluids.

When do I call my doctor or nurse?

• Call to make an appointment for your baby to be seen 1 week after you get home.

• Call if your baby looks yellow.

• Call if your baby has a fever (taken under the arm) of 100 degrees F or higher.

The First Few Days with Your Baby

- Call if your baby does not have 6 wet diapers in 24 hours.

- Call if your baby has pus, bleeding or a bad smell from the belly button.

- Call if you feel down or blue and do not feel like taking care of your baby.

- Call if you have questions about the care of your baby.

Word List

A

- **abuse**—Hurting or doing harm to a person.
- **accident**—To get hurt.
- **addicted**—When someone has a strong need or desire to do something like smoke or take drugs.
- **AIDS**—A disease passed by unprotected sex or IV drug users that causes bad sickness and death.
- **alcohol**—(1) Beer, wine, or drinks with hard liquor. (2) Another kind of alcohol, called rubbing alcohol, is put on the skin to keep it dry and clean. This alcohol is not for drinking.
- **amniotic sac**—This is a sac that grows inside the uterus. It holds the baby, the placenta, and a watery fluid called the amniotic fluid. It is often called the water bag. It protects the growing baby inside the uterus.
- **antacids**—Pills or liquid to help heartburn.
- **antibiotics**—Medicine ordered by a doctor to kill germs that cause infection.
- **anxious**—Worried or upset.
- **appetite**—A normal desire for food.
- **ashamed**—Feeling of shame, guilt, or disgrace.

Word List

B

- **belly button**—The place in the middle of the belly where the umbilical cord was attached.

- **birth control**—Things people do to prevent getting pregnant.

- **birth defects**—Physical or mental problems that babies are born with.

- **bladder**—The organ in the body that holds urine (pee).

- **bleeding**—Losing blood from the body.

- **blood pressure**—The force of the blood moving through the body measured with a cuff on the arm.

- **blood sugar**—The amount of sugar called glucose that is in the blood.

- **bottle feeding**—Feeding a baby using a bottle and nipple and formula bought from the store instead of your breast.

- **bowel**—The intestine also called the gut. A part of the body that food passes through and turns into solid waste.

- **bowel movement**—It is the way that we pass solid material (waste) from the body.

- **breastfeeding**—Feeding a baby using the breast instead of a bottle.

C

- **caffeine**—A drug found in coffee, tea, chocolate, and other food. It is a mild upper. A lot of caffeine is not good during pregnancy.

- **calories**—A measure of energy from food.

- **cervix**—The lower end or neck of the uterus. It opens into the vagina. The cervix opens wide during labor to let the baby out.

- **cesarean section (C-section)**—An operation done to remove a baby from the mother through the belly.

- **circumcision**—An operation done to remove the loose skin covering the tip of the penis of a new baby boy.

- **clots**—A rounded mass that is made of blood and other body tissue.

- **colostrum**—Early breast milk that is yellow and sticky.

- **community services**—Places that can help you or tell you where to get help for many things such as medical care, housing, food, work.

- **condom**—A latex cover put on a hard penis before sex. It prevents pregnancy and many sexually transmitted diseases.

- **constipation**—Hard, dry bowel movements that are hard to push out.

- **contraction**—The uterus gets tight and feels hard.

- **cooling down**—The time during exercise that you slow down before you stop.

- **cramps**—Belly pains.

D

- **delivery**—A baby being born.

- **diabetes**—A medical condition some women get during pregnancy caused by high sugar (glucose) in the blood.

Word List

- **diet**—To diet means eating less food in order to lose weight. A special diet means eating certain amounts and types of foods to help a medical condition.

- **disability benefits**—Money you get when you cannot work due to sickness or injury.

- **discomforts**—Having pain, feeling sick, or not feeling well.

- **dizzy**—Feeling like everything is spinning or turning around.

- **douche**—Water or other liquid put into the vagina to clean it.

- **drugs**—Something taken for sickness or disease. This is called medicine. Street drugs are taken to get high or feel good. These types of drugs are bad for people and unborn babies.

E

- **embryo**—This is what the baby is called during the first 8 weeks of growth in the mother's uterus.

- **episiotomy**—A cut made at the opening of the vagina during the delivery of the baby. It allows more room for the baby to come out.

- **exercise**—Being active and moving around. Body movement that makes the heart beat and breathing go faster.

F

- **fever**—The body is hotter than normal.

- **fiber**—Part of plants like fruits, vegetables, and grains that the body does not digest or use. Fiber helps people have regular bowel movements.

- **folate**—B vitamin also known as folic acid.
- **folic acid**—B vitamin needed in pregnancy and before a woman gets pregnant. It helps to prevent certain birth defects.
- **food cravings**—A strong desire to eat certain foods.
- **fumes**—Something in the air that is bad for you to breathe in.

G

- **glucose tolerance test**—A special test to see how much sugar or glucose is in your blood.

H

- **headache**—A pain in your head.
- **health insurance**—A company (also known as health plan) that pays or helps you pay for your health care. They may tell you where to go for health care.
- **healthy baby**—A baby that is born without health problems.
- **heartburn**—A burning feeling in your upper stomach.
- **heating pad**—An electric pad that feels warm.
- **hemorrhoids**—Swollen veins in and around the rectum.
- **herbs**—Plants used to make medicine.
- **high blood pressure**—The force of the blood moving through the body is higher than normal.
- **HIV**—The virus that causes AIDS.
- **hormones**—Chemicals made by the body to do certain things.

- **hot tubs**—A large tub that can hold a few people. It has hot water and jets that shoot out water.
- **humidifier**—A machine that puts a mist of water into the air.

I

- **infection**—Sickness caused by germs you cannot see. An infection can happen inside the body or on the skin.
- **iron**—Something found in foods that is good for the blood.

J

- **junk food**—Foods that are high in calories. They look and taste good but are not good for you or your baby.

K

- **Kegel exercises**—Exercises that make the muscles around your vagina strong and help you to hold urine (pee).
- **kick counts**—A way to keep track of how often your baby moves.

L

- **labor**—Contractions of the uterus that get harder and come often. They make the cervix open, which allows the baby to come out.
- **labor pains**—The pain that comes with contractions of the uterus.

M

- **mental retardation**—A birth defect that causes a baby to be slow to learn. This problem stays with a person all their life.

- **microwave**—A special oven that heats or cooks food or liquids very fast. Some parts can be very hot and burn a person. Do not warm a baby's bottle in a microwave.

- **miscarriage**—Loss of the baby from the uterus before the baby can live.

- **mist machine**—Same thing as a humidifier. You put water into it and it puts a mist of water into the air.

- **mood swings**—Feeling happy and then sad or angry in a short period of time.

- **morning sickness**—Feeling like throwing up during the first 3–4 months of pregnancy.

N

- **nausea**—A feeling like you have to throw up.

- **non-stress test**—A special test done to check the baby's heart rate when he moves.

P

- **pacifier**—A special nipple for babies to suck on that calms them.

- **Pap smear**—A test done to check for cervical cancer. Cells are taken from the cervix and tested.

- **pee**—Urine. Liquid waste from the body.

- **pelvic exam**—An exam by a doctor or nurse that checks the vagina, cervix, uterus, and other organs.

- **period**—The bloody discharge that comes out of a girl's vagina each month. This is called menstruation.

- **placenta**—It grows in the uterus of a pregnant woman. It is attached to the baby by the umbilical (belly-button) cord. The placenta supplies the baby with food. The placenta comes out after the baby is born. It is also called the afterbirth.

- **poison**—Something that makes you very sick if taken into the body.

- **pregnancy**—The time when a baby grows inside a woman.

- **pregnancy test**—A urine or blood test to tell if a woman is pregnant. A woman can buy a pregnancy test to do at home or have a test done at a doctor's office or health clinic.

- **prenatal**—The time before the baby is born.

- **pressure**—A feeling that something is pushing or pressing.

R

- **rectal**—Refers to the rectum.
- **rectum**—Where bowel movements come out.
- **relax**—Taking it easy or resting.
- **risks**—Things that can hurt your unborn baby.

Word List

S

- **second hand smoke**—Breathing in the smoke from a person who is smoking close to you.

- **sexually transmitted diseases (STDs)**—Diseases that can be passed through sex acts.

- **sitz bath**—Sitting in warm water to comfort and heal hemorrhoids or other problems in the rectum and vaginal area.

- **smoking**—Breathing smoke from a cigarette into the lungs.

- **snack**—Small amounts of food you eat between meals.

- **social worker**—A person trained to help people with problems like finding a doctor, paying bills, and finding a place to live.

- **sodium**—Another word for salt. Too much sodium makes the body hold water.

- **speculum**—A special tool doctors use to hold open the vagina while doing a pap test.

- **stress test**—A special test done in the hospital to check the baby's heart beat during contractions of the uterus.

- **stretches**—Gets bigger.

- **support groups**—More than three people who have the same problems. They get together to talk and try to help each other.

- **support hose**—Tight stockings that help the blood flow in your legs.

- **swell**—To get bigger.

T

- **temperature**—How hot something is.

U

- **ultrasound**—A test done in a doctor's office or clinic that shows a picture of the baby growing in the uterus.
- **umbilical cord**—It connects the baby to the placenta. The cord brings food to the baby from the mother through the placenta. It takes away waste products from the baby. The umbilical cord is cut after the baby is born. The part that is left becomes the belly button.
- **unemployment**—Not working.
- **uterus**—This is the organ in a woman that carries a growing baby. The muscle of the uterus stretches as the baby grows.

V

- **vagina**—The last passage that the baby goes through during birth.
- **varicose veins**—Swelling of the veins in the legs.
- **vitamins**—Pills or liquid your doctor tells you to take during pregnancy. Vitamins help a woman to have a healthy baby.
- **virus**—Something too small to see that can pass from one person to another and make you sick. A virus cannot be cured by antibiotics.
- **vomiting**—Throwing up.

Word List

W

- **warning signs**—Things that you feel or see that are not normal. They are a sign that something may be wrong.

X

- **x-rays**—A picture taken using low doses of radiation. It's important to avoid x-rays during pregnancy.

What's in This Book from A to Z

What's in This Book from A to Z

What's in This Book from A to Z

People We Want to Thank

We want to thank the following people for their help with this book.

Angela Maria Acevedo, RN

Kristina Adame

Albert Barnett, MD

Mary Martha Bernadett, MD, MBA

Laura Blank, RN, MSN, CNS

Mary Bell

Tracey Fremd, NP

Cristina Garibay

Ruth Goldenberg, MD

Sandy Harbour, CNM

Gino Hasler

Sharon Mann-Johnson

Amy Jones

Neil C. Jouvenat, MD

Elda Juarez

Lilia Knudtson, RN, CNP, MSN

Mitzi Krockover, MD

Rita London

Victor London

J. Kelly Mantis, MD

Thomas R. Mayer, MD

Christel McRae, RN, PHN

Patricia Meili

Chawn Naughton

Linda Nixon, RN, CNM, MSN

Irene Diane Nunez

Doriann Oravec

Diane Patton, MD

Steven Rosenberg, MD, MPH

Araceli Ramirez

Nancy Rushton, RN, BSN

Marian Ryan, RRT, MPH, CHES

Ann Santos

Justin Segal

Michael Villaire

Alexandra L. Vreugdenhil, LVN

Elaine M. Weiner, RN, MPH

Carolyn Wendt

Dianne Woo

Sara Ye

Margaret Zickrick

Notes

Other Books in the Series

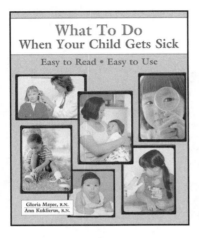

ISBN 978-0-9701245-0-0
$12.95

What To Do
When Your Child Gets Sick*

There are many things you can do at home for your child. At last, an easy to read, easy to use book written by two nurses who know. This book tells you:

- What to look for when your child is sick.
- When to call the doctor.
- How to take your child's temperature.
- What to do when your child has the flu.
- How to care for cuts and scrapes.
- What to feed your child when he or she is sick.
- How to stop the spread of infection.
- How to prevent accidents around your home.
- What to do in an emergency.

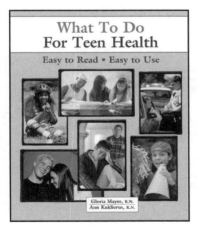

ISBN 978-0-9701245-2-4
$12.95

What To Do
For Teen Health

The teen years are hard on parents and teens. There are many things you can do to help your teen. At last, an easy to read, easy to use book written by two nurses. This book tells you:

- About the body changes that happen to teens.
- How to get ready for the teen years.
- How to talk with your teen.
- What you can do to feel closer to your teen.
- How to help your teen do well in school.
- All about dating and sex.
- How to keep your teen safe.
- The signs of trouble and where to go for help.

Also available in Spanish.
*Also available in Vietnamese, Chinese, and Korean.
To order, call (800) 434-4633.

Other Books in the Series

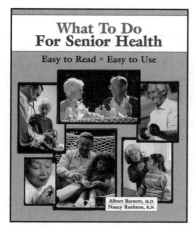

ISBN 978-0-9701245-4-8
$12.95

What To Do
For Senior Health*

There are many things that you can do to take charge of your health during your senior years. This book tells about:

- Body changes that come with aging.
- Common health problems of seniors.
- Things to consider about health insurance.
- How to choose a doctor and where to get health care.
- Buying and taking medicines.
- Simple things you can do to prevent falls and accidents.
- What you can do to stay healthy.

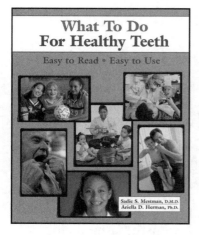

ISBN 978-0-9720148-0-9
$12.95

What To Do
For Healthy Teeth

It is important to take good care of your teeth from an early age. This book tells how to do that. It also explains all about teeth, gums, and how dentists work with you to keep your teeth healthy.

- How to care for your teeth and gums.
- What you need to care for your teeth and gums.
- Caring for your teeth when you're having a baby.
- Caring for your child's teeth.
- When to call the dentist.
- What to expect at a dental visit.
- Dental care needs for seniors.
- What to do if you hurt your mouth or teeth.

Also available in Spanish.
*Also available in Vietnamese.
To order, call (800) 434-4633.

Other Books in the Series

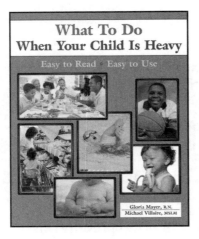

ISBN 978-0-9721048-4-7
$12.95

What To Do When Your Child Is Heavy

There are many things you can do to help your heavy child live a healthy lifestyle. Here's an easy to read, easy to use book that tells you:

- How to tell if your child is heavy.
- How to shop and pay for healthy food.
- Dealing with your heavy child's feelings and self-esteem.
- How to read the Nutrition Facts Label.
- Healthy breakfasts, lunches and dinners.
- Correct portion sizes.
- Why exercise is so important.
- Tips for eating healthy when you eat out.
- Information on diabetes and other health problems of heavy children.

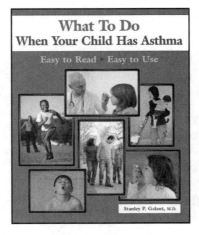

ISBN 978-0-9720148-6-1
$12.95

What To Do When Your Child Has Asthma

Having a child with asthma can be scary. This easy to read, easy to use book tells you what you can do to help your child deal with asthma:

- How to tell if your child needs help right away.
- Signs that your child has asthma.
- Triggers for an asthma attack.
- Putting together an Asthma Action Plan.
- How to use a peak flow meter.
- The different kinds of asthma medicine.
- How to talk to your child's day care and teachers about your child's asthma.
- Making sure your child gets enough exercise.
- Helping your child to take their asthma medicine the right way.
- What to do for problems like upset stomach, hay fever and stuffy nose.

Also available in Spanish.
To order, call (800) 434-4633.